Eat Well & Exercise

Harnessing Today's Top Anti-Aging Formula

2022 Report

A Special Report published by
the editors of *Tufts Health & Nutrition Letter*
in cooperation with
The Gerald J. and Dorothy R. Friedman School of Nutrition Science and Policy
Tufts University

Eat Well & Exercise: Harnessing Today's Top Anti-Aging Formula

Medical Editor: Roger A. Fielding, Ph.D., Associate Center Director and Senior Scientist, Jean Mayer USDA Human Nutrition Research Center on Aging, Professor of Nutrition, Gerald J. and Dorothy R. Friedman School of Nutrition Science and Policy at Tufts University, Professor of Medicine, Tufts University School of Medicine

Author: Marsha McCulloch, MS, RDN
Update Author: JoAnn Milivojevic
Belvoir Editor: Cindy Foley
Creative Director, Belvoir Media Group: Judi Crouse
Production: Mary Francis McGavic

Publisher, Belvoir Media Group: Timothy H. Cole
Executive Editor, Book Division, Belvoir Media Group: Lynn Russo

Print ISBN 978-1-879620-68-1
Digital ISBN 978-1-879620-73-5

To order additional copies of this report or for customer-service questions, please call 877-300-0253 or write: Health Special Reports, 535 Connecticut Avenue, Norwalk, CT 06854-1713. To subscribe to the monthly newsletter *Tufts Health & Nutrition Letter,* call 800-274-7581 or write to the address above.

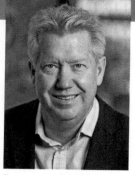

Roger A. Fielding, PhD
Associate Center
Director and Senior
Scientist, Jean
Mayer USDA Human
Nutrition Research
Center on Aging
Professor of Nutrition,
Gerald J. and Dorothy
R. Friedman School
of Nutrition Science
and Policy at Tufts
University
Professor of Medicine,
Tufts University
School of Medicine

As our country and the world emerge from the COVID-19 pandemic, we look forward to the restoration of our normal way of living and reflecting on a changed world, hopeful for the future. With a sense of renewal, we now can envision a new and better way of living that embraces evidence-based healthy lifestyles with sensible food choices, mindfulness, and participation in regular physical activity. As we continue to find lifestyle interventions that help us extend our "health-span," let's also reflect on the many opportunities that await us in the future. It is my hope that we rise from the pandemic stronger than before.

The message to eat well and exercise remains, but each year additional evidence is discovered that further reinforces these important components of good health. We need to address prolonging health-span as life expectancy continues to rise. With emerging challenges to our health-care system that were revealed during the pandemic, we must re-double our efforts to promote healthy aging, which is the key to sustained resilience to multiple environmental stressors, including infectious diseases and other harmful agents. All the while, we need to make sure that our new knowledge embraces diversity and inclusion and that we ensure access to the health benefits of proper nutrition and regular physical activity to all people.

I hope you enjoy reading about the most recent research illustrating the benefits of diet and physical activity on healthy and active aging. Every year, additional evidence suggests that these lifestyle behaviors are bridges to maintaining our independence and aging successfully. Importantly, it's never too late to make healthy lifestyle changes to benefit our functioning, and these effects can be achieved regardless of chronological age. Remember, small changes can have big impacts.

Roger A. Fielding, PhD

TABLE OF CONTENTS

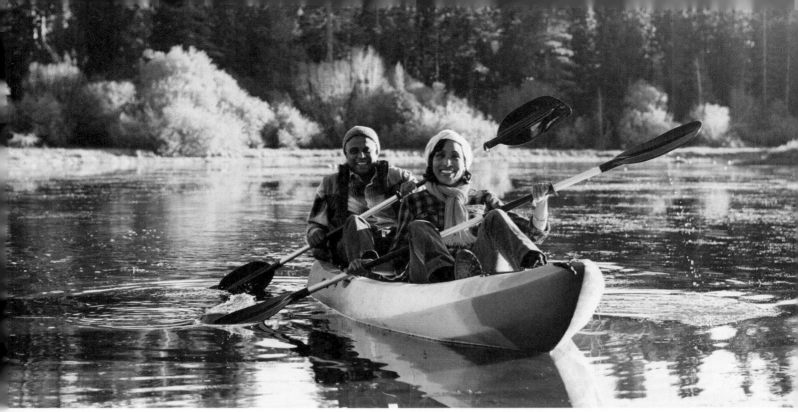

© Monkeybusinessimages | Dreamstime

New Findings

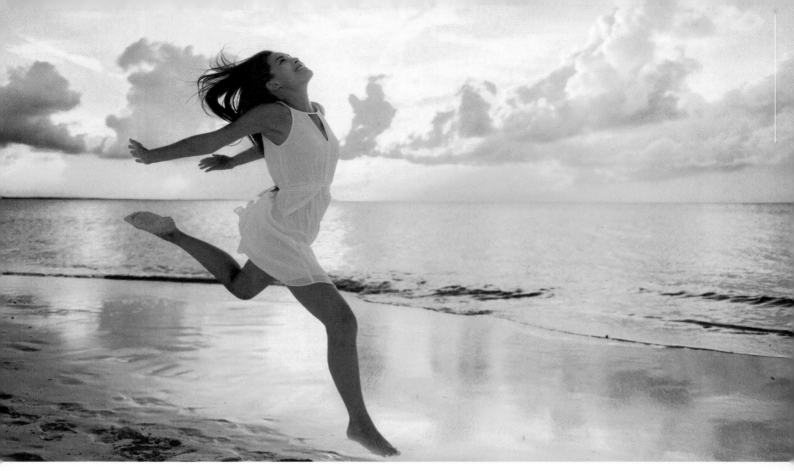

© Martinmark | Dreamstime

Eating well and being physically active can improve how you feel, think, and move every day. The combination gives you a better quality of life and happiness.

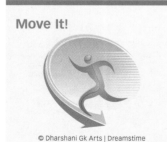

Move It!

© Dharshani Gk Arts | Dreamstime

More Powerful Than a Drug

As miraculous as medications may be, they cannot overcome the effects of a sedentary lifestyle and a nutrient-poor diet. Your well-being is in your own hands.

1 Optimum Wellness

If you had to name just two things that could profoundly affect quality of life, what would you say? Of course, given the title of this Special Health Report gives you the answer: eat well and exercise. Why, then, do so many people struggle to do so? The answers are numerous and complex. But some solutions may be easier than you think. These pages are filled with evidence-based recommendations and insights that will motivate you to overcome obstacles to help you feel and look your best.

The concept of nutritious food and daily physical activity to improve overall well-being is not new. But how do food and movement advance quality of life? Researchers are constantly on the hunt to substantiate what most people intuit to be true. For example, a 2019 study at the Jean Mayer USDA Human Nutrition Research Center on Aging at Tufts, published in *Experimental Gerontology*, sought to know if the composition of the gut microbiome had any influence on physical functioning. The gut microbiome refers to microorganisms that naturally live in your gastrointestinal tract. The microbiome consists of trillions of bacteria, fungi, and viruses—all of which combine in a complex and typically symbiotic way. In simple terms, when the microbes are in balance, the gut is healthy and happy. When out of balance, an unhappy gut communicates through aches, pains, gas, bloat, and other symptoms.

What we eat and drink greatly determine the contents of the gut microbiome. In that study, Tufts researchers compared gut bacteria from 18 older physically high-functioning adults with favorable body composition (higher percentage of lean mass, lower percentage of fat mass) with 11 physically low-functioning older adults with less favorable body composition. Bacterial differences were found between the two groups. Similar differences were found when mice were colonized with bacterial samples from the two human groups. While a study with mice doesn't prove anything in humans, it shows promise for the future. Researchers discovered that grip strength was increased in mice colonized with samples from the high-functioning older human adults. This suggests that the gut microbiome plays a role in mechanisms related to muscle strength in older adults.

Foods that support a healthy microbiome, such as prebiotic and probiotic foods, are smart choices. And they are the same foods recommended for good overall health and immune system support (see "Prebiotic and Probiotic Foods"). By optimizing your diet with these foods, you give your immune system a fighting chance to overcome infections, including from viruses that cause influenza and COVID-19. Similarly, maintaining a healthy weight supports your immune system. Excessive body fat is inflammatory, and obesity has been implicated as a risk factor for COVID-19 and other diseases (see "Obesity Lowers Immunity").

Of course, human life also benefits from medications, such as with drugs that can help control life-threatening diseases like diabetes, hypertension (elevated blood pressure), and hyperlipidemia (high cholesterol). But as miraculous as these medications may be, they cannot overcome the effects of a sedentary lifestyle and a nutrient-poor diet.

A Pound of Prevention

The past few years have taught us how critical it is to our health to maintain a healthy immune system, which is significantly strengthened by a nutritious diet and regular physical activity. Researchers discovered that consistently meeting exercise guidelines of at least 150 minutes per week reduced severe COVID-19 outcomes ("Exercise Reduces COVID-19 Severity").

The dynamic duo of diet and exercise helps prevent illnesses, speeds healing, supports cardiovascular health, preserves muscle function, improves mood, and helps keep your brain sharp and your bones strong. That's an incredible list of benefits.

Smart food and exercise choices reduce the risk for early death and may lower the hazards

Prebiotic and Probiotic Foods

Prebiotic foods contain a type of fiber that feeds the friendly bacteria in your gut. They include asparagus, bananas, garlic, Jerusalem artichokes, onions, soybeans, and wheat. Probiotic foods contain live bacteria. These foods include plain yogurt with live cultures, kefir, and fermented products such as sauerkraut, kimchi, kombucha tea, and unpasteurized pickles and vegetables. Both these categories of foods help support a healthy gut microbiome and your immune system.

NEW FINDING

Obesity Lowers Immunity

According to a study from the University of Michigan, obesity likely triggers the immune system to react to a COVID-19 infection in way that makes it difficult to fight off the virus. This conclusion was based on an analysis of numerous existing studies on inflammation, immunity, and obesity. People with obesity and metabolic disease (such as diabetes or fatty liver) frequently experience a state of low-grade chronic inflammation, which impairs their ability to fight off infections. Researchers specifically noted that among patients ages 19 to 64 admitted to the hospital with COVID-19, those with pre-existing conditions caused by excessive body fat, which was defined as a high body mass index (BMI) were more likely to be admitted to intensive care. Though older adults are more vulnerable to viral infection, younger adults are more likely to have a higher BMI than older people, which increases younger adults' susceptibility to severe COVID-19 illness. The same appears to be true of young children with obesity, as they, too, were more vulnerable to severe COVID-19 reactions, compared to normal-weight children. Researchers say more research into the mechanisms and pathways altered by excessive fat is critical to understanding disease severity and the possible treatments for COVID-19 and other diseases.
Endocrinology, Sept. 3, 2020

NEW FINDING

Exercise Reduces COVID-19 Severity

Sedentary people infected with the novel coronavirus (SARS-CoV-2) that causes COVID-19 disease had a greater risk of hospitalization, admission to the intensive care unit (ICU), and death compared to infected people who were consistently meeting recommended exercise guidelines. This conclusion was based upon analyzing data from 48,440 adults with a COVID-19 diagnosis between January 2020 and October 2020. Researchers gathered self-reported exercise data over a two-year period (March 2018 to March 2020). They linked each person's physical activity category (consistently inactive = 0–10 min/week, some activity = 11–149 min/week, consistently meeting guidelines = 150+ min/week) to the risk of hospitalization, ICU admission, and death after COVID-19 diagnosis. The study reported that consistent exercise (at least 150 minutes per week of moderate physical activity) was strongly associated with reduced risk for severe COVID-19 illness. The researchers recommend that public-health agencies step up to more diligently promote physical activity and call for exercise recommendations to be a part of routine medical care.
British Sports Journal, March 30, 2021

of such chronic diseases as high blood pressure, stroke, type 2 diabetes, heart disease, and even some cancers. If you already have a chronic condition, healthful dietary choices and physical activity may help you manage it better, and in some cases, eliminate the need for medications.

According to the most recent Physical Activity Guidelines for Americans Advisory Committee Report to the U.S. Department of Health and Human Services, some conditions are less common among individuals who are, or become, more physically active. In addition, people with some of these conditions who are more physically active have improved physical function and a better quality of life. They benefit from a reduced risk of premature death, a lowered risk of developing other chronic diseases or conditions, and a decreased risk of progression of the disease they already have (see "Defense Against Diabetes" and "Cancer Risk Reduction").

Being active decreases anxiety, improves sleep and some brain functions, and increases quality of life. Even small amounts of activity help. Even less than 48 minutes per week of physical activity could reduce the risk of physical disability in many older adults (see "Simple Swaps").

Protection for the Heart

The best weapons against heart disease (in addition to quitting or never having smoked) are diet and exercise. For evidence that diet and exercise recommendations really work, a 2018 study led by a Tufts University researcher investigated the association between circulating blood levels of n-3 polyunsaturated fatty acids (n-PUFAs) and healthy aging among older adults (average age 74). The researchers found that 89 percent of the participants experienced unhealthy aging over the 23-year study period, while 11 percent experienced healthy aging, which was defined as survival free of major chronic diseases and without mental or physical dysfunction.

Defense Against Diabetes

According to the National Diabetes Statistics Report from the Centers for Disease Control and Prevention, about 44 percent of Americans over age 18 are living with diabetes or prediabetes. The percentage of people with this life-threatening condition increases with age. Diet and exercise have been proven to reduce the risk of developing diabetes and are a key part of treatment for those living with this condition.

An intriguing 2019 study published in *Cell Metabolism* investigated a form of intermittent fasting called early time-restricted feeding. Study outcomes showed that eating all meals by mid-afternoon and fasting the rest of the day improved blood sugar control, blood pressure, and oxidative stress, even when people didn't change what they ate. Eating early in the day may be a particularly beneficial form of intermittent fasting because the body's ability to keep blood sugar under control is better in the morning than it is in the afternoon and the evening.

A healthy diet can help with weight loss and keep blood sugar levels under control, and physical activity makes muscles more sensitive to insulin, which further helps to control blood sugar. Evidence suggests that compared to a sedentary lifestyle, even low levels of physical activity can enhance insulin sensitivity and help reduce diabetes risk.

Cancer Risk Reduction

One-third of the cancer deaths in the United States each year are linked to poor diet, physical inactivity, and being overweight. Physical activity alone is believed to reduce the risk of developing cancer of the breast, colon, bladder, endometrium, esophagus, kidney, lung, and stomach. While medical experts agree that physical activity can positively affect cancer treatment and recovery, what if you haven't been diligent about working out before a diagnosis? Will it matter now? The short answer is yes. And it's backed up by a comprehensive analysis of more than 2,000 studies.

A group of 40 experts from various organizations worldwide conducted a thorough review of studies that provided evidence on the positive effects of exercise in helping people prevent, manage, and recover from cancer. The evidence-backed recommendations, coordinated through the American College of Sports Medicine, calls for incorporating exercise into prevention and treatment plans. Researchers found that exercise lowers the risk of seven common types of cancer: colon, breast, endometrial, kidney, bladder, esophageal, and stomach. For cancer survivors, researchers recommend exercising during and after cancer treatment to decrease fatigue, anxiety, and depression and to improve physical function and quality of life.

Healthy dietary patterns provide nutrients and compounds that might help deactivate carcinogens, turn on tumor-suppressor genes, and affect cell growth. Less healthful choices, like red and processed meats (for example, hot dogs, sausage, and bacon), have been shown to increase cancer risk.

Maintaining a healthy weight through good food choices and activity also is an important anti-cancer strategy, since excess weight and obesity are linked to the risk for at least 13 cancers.

While many factors, including genetics and environment, play a role in the development of chronic illness, following the advice in this Special Health Report can give your body the tools it needs to stay as healthy as possible and to fight against or better manage whatever comes your way.

The researchers found the healthy-aging group had higher levels of n-PUFAs. A possible explanation for this effect is that n-PUFAs help regulate blood pressure, heart rate, and inflammation.

Doctors have long been aware that arteries thicken and harden as we age due to the buildup of plaques. They used to think that plaque built up over a lifetime, like rings on a tree. Now they know that inflammation irritates the vascular endothelium (the lining of the blood vessels) and causes plaque to grow. Controlling inflammation, high cholesterol, high blood pressure, high triglycerides, and obesity by following diet and exercise tips like the ones presented in this Special Health Report can help protect your blood vessels from that damaging irritation.

Research shows that the higher a person's level of physical fitness, the less likely he or she is to die prematurely from cardiovascular disease. Based on this data, all major cardiovascular medical societies have made physical activity a key part of guidelines to prevent cardiovascular disease. Small changes to your diet also may be enough to improve your heart health. The American Heart Association suggestions include:

Enjoy More:
- fruits
- vegetables
- whole grains
- poultry
- fish
- nuts
- low-fat dairy products

Limit Intake of:
- red meat
- saturated fat
- trans fat
- sodium
- high-calorie/low-nutrient foods
- sugary foods and beverages

A Healthy, Happy Life
Your physical, mental, emotional, and social functioning make up what researchers call your "health-related quality of life." Eating well and exercising add to your health-related quality of life by working to keep you in good health and by supporting the strength, energy, and mental capacity you need to live a full, satisfying, and productive long life.

Staying Strong
Age-related muscle loss, called sarcopenia, is a natural part of the aging process and begins in the third decade of life. After age 30, people can lose from 3 to 5 percent of muscle mass per decade. If nothing is done to counterbalance this consequence of aging, it can lead to frailty, obesity, and loss of mobility.

Age-related muscle weakness dramatically increases the risk of falling, and falls are another big reason older people must leave their homes for long-term-care facilities. Half of the accidental deaths among people ages 65 and older are related to falls. Many people admitted to long-term-care facilities need to be there because they can no longer perform activities of daily living (like eating, bathing, dressing, and walking).

But muscle can be rebuilt at any age. A series of landmark studies published in the 1990s highlighted the profound role progressive resistance training can have on increasing muscle mass, muscle size, and functional capacity in older adults. In one of those studies, participants ages 90 to 99 increased their mid-thigh muscle strength, on average, 174 percent.

It is essential to strength train at least twice per week. Whether it's resistance bands, barbells, or body weight doesn't matter. What does matter is exhausting a muscle through repetition or load—because muscle builds when it's pushed out of its comfort zone. See Chapter 2 for details on resistance training.

Muscle makes up more than half of typical body mass, and it does more than just move our bodies and make us strong. Important chemical reactions take place in muscle cells, which is part of the reason muscle loss can lead to

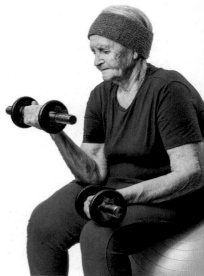

© Photobac | Dreamstime

Muscles can be strengthened at any age.

insulin resistance (a precursor of diabetes) and may be involved in the development of high cholesterol and high triglycerides, markers of cardiovascular disease.

Reduce Muscle Loss. Disease, inflammation, and age-related changes at the cellular level can all contribute to sarcopenia, but a lack of activity and poor nutrition also are major contributing factors. Even sedentary older adults can significantly reduce disability through relatively small increases in regular participation in physical activity. So, while everyone loses some muscle over time, a healthy diet and regular physical activity can reduce the rate of loss.

Muscle is built from protein, and bones rely on dietary nutrients like calcium, vitamin D, and magnesium, so eating a balanced diet is essential. But beware of supplements making bold promises.

A 2018 study published in the *Journal of Nutrition* found that consuming protein supplements did not help active older men build more muscle or gain more strength than resistance exercise training alone. Forty-one men with an average age of 70 completed whole-body resistance training three times a week for 12 weeks. Half the group drank a supplement containing 21 grams of protein after exercise and every night before bed. The other half drank a beverage with the same number of calories but no protein. At the end of the study, both groups were able to lift more weight and tests showed increased muscle mass, but the protein group did not improve any more than the placebo group.

Brain Benefits

Your cognitive ability can fall prey to reduced blood flow to the brain, loss of gray matter, and the buildup of sticky tangles and plaques of certain proteins. But physical activity and good nutrition can help you fight back.

As the brain ages, the number and size of its blood vessels shrink, leaving fewer alternate routes for blood to take if some vessels are narrowed or damaged by stroke. A heart-healthy diet can help keep blood vessels clear, and regular aerobic exercise can increase the number of blood vessels in your brain, even if you don't start until middle age. Studies show that people who lead more active lifestyles had less loss of brain matter than their less-active peers.

Diet matters, too. The Mediterranean diet, which relies heavily on fruit, fish, vegetables, and olive oil, may increase brain volume and lower the risk of mild cognitive decline and Alzheimer's disease. Omega-3 fatty acids, antioxidants, and certain B vitamins are thought to be especially good for preserving brain health. But strive to get these nutrients in food. Evidence is lacking in whether nutritional supplements play a protective role.

Preserving cognitive function is essential, but keeping your vision sharp is important to enjoying your golden years, too. Vitamins C and E, beta-carotene, zinc, and the plant compounds lutein and zeaxanthin are important weapons in the fight against blindness. Experts recommend you eat fish at least twice a week to support eye health.

Consequences of Inactivity

Inactivity ranks alongside tobacco, alcohol, and obesity as a leading cause of reduced healthy life expectancy. Beyond thinking about including formal exercise in your routine, a growing body of evidence suggests it is just as important to look for ways to simply sit less during

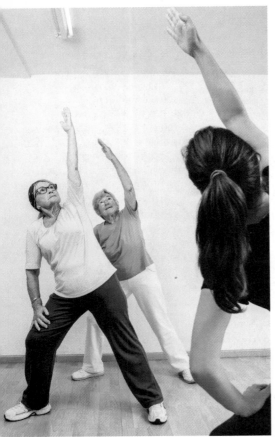
© Karelnoppe | Dreamstime

Regular aerobic exercise helps to increase the number of blood vessels in the brain and throughout the body.

the day (see "Avoid Inactivity to Improve Life Quality").

Research suggests that people who sit a lot and don't exercise regularly are likely at the greatest risk of chronic disease and premature death. However, even if you have a regular workout routine and meet the minimum physical-activity guidelines, sitting too much the rest of the time can take a toll on your health, increasing the risk of obesity, type 2 diabetes, cardiovascular disease, and certain cancers. For a look at the health impacts of a sedentary lifestyle versus an active lifestyle, see "Boost Your Health Benefits with an Active Lifestyle."

Preventing and managing chronic diseases, staying strong, and staying mentally sharp all extend the "health-span" of your life. That fountain of youth we all wish for comes from eating well and exercising regularly.

Boost Your Health Benefits with an Active Lifestyle

Based on available studies, this chart compares sedentary older adults to active older adults who engage in regular physical activity, including aerobic exercise and resistance training.

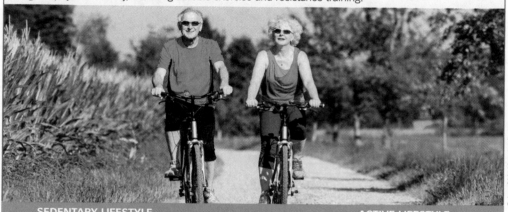

© Arne9001 | Dreamstime

SEDENTARY LIFESTYLE		ACTIVE LIFESTYLE
• accelerated loss of muscle mass and strength	**muscle strength**	• prevention or slowing of muscle loss and increase in muscle strength
• decrease in bone density	**bone density**	• bone loss slowed or prevented, with potential increase in bone density
• blood vessels stiffen and blood pressure rises	**blood pressure**	• blood vessels expand more easily, resulting in lower blood pressure
• higher blood sugar	**blood-sugar control**	• muscles become more sensitive to insulin, helping to lower blood sugar
• decrease in HDL (good) cholesterol	**cholesterol**	• increase in HDL (good) cholesterol
• fat accumulates more readily in the abdomen and triggers inflammation and insulin resistance	**abdominal obesity**	• less abdominal fat
• women: 1,600 • men: 2,000	**average daily calorie needs**	• women: 1,800–2,200 • men: 2,200–2,800
• decrease in resting metabolism	**metabolism**	• increase in resting metabolism • better able to use fat as fuel
• lower sleep efficiency	**sleep efficiency** (time actually asleep after falling asleep)	• higher sleep efficiency
• higher risk of cognitive decline	**brain function**	• lower risk of cognitive decline
• lose ability to maintain independent living earlier	**independence**	• prolonged ability to maintain independent living

NEW FINDING

Avoid Inactivity to Improve Life Quality

It isn't just what you do, it's what you don't do that impacts quality of life, according to research led from the Department of Kinesiology at Iowa State University. For their study, researchers wanted to know what would happen if people reallocated their time spent on physical activity, sedentary behavior, and sleep. A few small changes, as it turned out, garnered some meaningful results. Reallocating just 30 minutes from being inactive to light activity, or moderately activity to more high-intensity activity was associated with higher quality of life. Whereas shifting time away from moderate or intense physical activity toward lighter activity, sedentary behavior, or sleep was associated with lower quality of life. The authors further concluded that short- and long-term psychological benefits may result from transitioning sedentary time to light physical activity, whereas increasing moderate-to-vigorous physical activity may be required to influence physical health.

American Journal of Preventive Medicine, May 2020

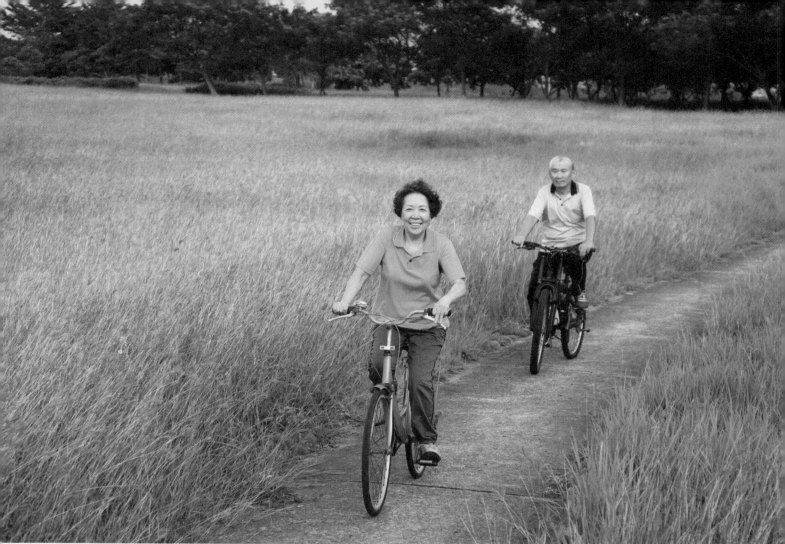

Being physically active with others can boost spirits, strengthen relationships, and improve overall well-being.

2 The Healing Power of Exercise

The extraordinary benefits of physical activity can't be over-emphasized. Life—human, animal, or insect—depends upon movement. Electrical impulses activate the heart. Brain cells communicate through chemicals that literally jump across space to reach receptors. Eyes blink, hair grows, and skin sheds and replenishes. Bodies are designed to move inside and out, and research has shown how miraculous activity can be. Even just a little dedicated exercise can reduce blood pressure, improve sleep, and quell anxiety.

It's little wonder then that exercise is such an extremely effective way to prevent disease, reduce symptoms, and even heal from traumas. Physical therapy following an accident or surgical procedure is widely prescribed by physicians and covered by most insurance—because therapeutic movement helps heal. And now more and more physicians recognize how powerful physical conditioning can be *before* a procedure.

Pre-habilitation is the term used for preparing the body before entering an operating room. It's common for those about to undergo knee or hip surgery to spend several weeks strengthening the supporting muscles of the joints being replaced. But pre-habilitation also has been shown to be beneficial prior to chemotherapy and before cardiovascular and abdominal surgeries to help people recover faster. A 2019 study published in the *Journal of the American College of Surgeons* compared patients in 21 hospitals in Michigan and found that pre-habilitation patients across the state left the hospital one day earlier and were more likely to go straight home rather than to a skilled nursing facility, compared with similar patients at the same hospital. Total costs for all care up to three months after surgery were nearly $3,200 less on average for those who went through pre-hab. Researchers say that pre-hab's physical training may work partly because it empowers the patient to engage in their own recovery, adding that patient empowerment is the "secret sauce" and harnessing it offers multiple benefits.

Exercise need not be expensive or complicated. You can do it at home, and just 30 minutes a day can make a difference. Building the exercise habit isn't always easy, but once the habit is formed, you may be surprised how much you look forward to that time to yourself. You may even feel dissatisfied if you miss a session because in a relatively short period of time most people realize how much better it feels to live in a body that is more fit and flexible.

Devote time and attention to physical fitness and the mind is sharper, the body moves more gracefully and painlessly, and emotions are better balanced. That's true whether you are a toddler or an elder. The general exercise recommendations don't change that much through the decades, but the particulars can help keep you motivated and safer while working out. Consider that just one session of moderate-to-vigorous physical activity can help:

- reduce blood pressure
- improve insulin sensitivity
- improve sleep
- reduce anxiety symptoms
- lead to clearer thinking on the day it is performed

Adopting a new physical activity routine and keeping it up can:

- decrease risk of certain cancers
- improve physical function among individuals of all ages
- decrease dementia risk
- prevent excessive weight gain
- improve perceived quality of life
- reduce the risk of clinical depression and reduce depression symptoms

Types of Exercise

The amount of exercise you need continues to be debated and researched, but the U.S. Department of Health and Human Services issues physical-activity guidelines based on this latest scientific information. These guidelines are updated every 10 years, and the most recent recommendations were released in 2018.

All adults should get 150 to 300 minutes a week of moderate-intensity aerobic exercise, which is less than 22 to 44 minutes per day (2½ to five hours per week). If you can step up the pace, vigorous-intensity exercise can help you reach your activity goals more quickly. Seventy-five minutes (1¼ hours) of vigorous aerobic activity is equivalent to 150 minutes of moderate-intensity activity (see "Defining Aerobic Exercise").

In addition to aerobic activity, experts recommend resistance training (muscle-strengthening exercises) for all adults,

© Dharshani Gk Arts | Dreamstime

Full-Body Emphasis

Try to work each major muscle group—think arms, shoulders, chest, abdomen, back, hips, and legs—at least twice a week.

Defining Aerobic Exercise

Although exercise intensity is relative, this chart gives you a general idea of what is commonly considered moderate or vigorous aerobic activity.

MODERATE INTENSITY		VIGOROUS INTENSITY	
• ballroom dancing	• shuffleboard	• aerobic dancing/	• race walking
• baseball or softball	• skiing, moderate	step aerobics	• rowing
• bicycling (< 10 mph)	(downhill or	• backpacking	• shoveling snow
• bowling	alpine)	• bicycling (> 10 mph)	• snowshoeing
• fishing and	• tai chi	• circuit or interval	• skiing, intense
hunting	• tennis (doubles)	training	(downhill or alpine)
• golf (without cart)	• walking briskly on	• cross-country	• soccer
• juggling	a level surface	skiing	• swimming laps
• kayaking	• water aerobics	• ice skating	• tennis (singles)
• mopping/	• yardwork	• jogging or running	• water (aqua)
vacuuming	(general)	• jumping rope	jogging
• shooting baskets	• yoga	• karate/kick boxing	• yardwork (heavy)

but particularly older adults. Aim to work each major muscle group (arms, shoulders, chest, abdomen, back, hips, and legs) at least twice a week.

Remember that the best exercise activity varies from person to person, based on individual goals and abilities. The most important thing is to find an exercise routine that you enjoy and are likely to maintain. Whether you're just getting started or looking to step up your exercise plan, slowly increase the amount of time you exercise then gradually increase the intensity (see "Safety When Exercising").

Heart-Healthy Exercise

Sometimes called endurance or cardiovascular exercise, aerobic activity involves moving large muscle groups in a rhythmic manner for an extended time. Common examples are brisk walking, dancing, swimming, jogging, and biking. Aerobic exercise enhances the performance of your heart, circulatory system, lungs, and muscles, so you may have more stamina and reduced risk factors for chronic disease, such as elevated blood pressure, cholesterol, and triglycerides. A large study published in the *Journal of the American College of Cardiology* in 2018 showed that going for a walk just a few times a week could protect you from developing heart failure.

With vigorous exercise, you get similar health benefits in half the time it takes you with moderate exercise. For example, 15 minutes of vigorous walking (such as walking up hills) is equivalent to 30 minutes of moderate-intensity walking. A particularly vigorous form of exercise that has been shown to have tremendous health benefits is high-intensity interval training (HIIT).

HIIT has been used to train athletes for many years, but recently has grown in popularity among the general public. HIIT workouts involve repeated bouts of high-intensity effort, with recovery time between each bout. They improve both aerobic and anaerobic fitness, blood pressure, cardiovascular health, insulin sensitivity, and cholesterol profiles, and reduce abdominal fat and body weight while maintaining muscle mass. Part of the appeal of HIIT workouts is that you get all the benefits of continuous-endurance workouts in a shorter period of time. HIIT training can be modified easily for people of all fitness levels, and it works with any kind of exercise, from walking, biking, or swimming to elliptical, cross-training, and group exercise classes.

The intense workout periods push your heart rate to 80 to 95 percent of your estimated maximum heart rate. The recovery periods typically last at least as long as the work periods and usually are performed at 40 to 50 percent of your estimated maximum heart rate. A HIIT session can last from 20 to 60 minutes. During the high-intensity interval, you should be able to carry on a conversation, but with difficulty. The recovery interval should feel comfortable.

The ratio of exercise to recovery can vary, but 1:1 is typical. For example, you may perform three minutes of hard work followed by a three-minute recovery period of low-intensity activity. High-intensity bouts should not last more than eight minutes. Another popular HIIT training protocol is the "spring interval training method," which involves 30 seconds of near full-out effort followed by 4 to 4½ minutes of recovery, repeated three to five times. HIIT workouts exhaust your body. One session a week, complemented by regular "steady state" endurance workouts, is probably enough. You can work your way up to two HIIT sessions a week but be sure to spread them out to give your body the extra time it needs to recover from this intense exercise.

If you are typically sedentary, older, or haven't been doing much physical activity, it's recommended that you start with a consultation with your physician. If you get the go-ahead from your doctor, you'll need to build a base fitness level before beginning HIIT training. Consistent aerobic training (three to five times a week for 20 to 60 minutes per session at moderate-to-high intensity) for several weeks will get your muscles ready for interval training. This also will give you the proper exercise form and muscle strength you need to reduce the risk of injury.

Need to Start Easier? Walking is a great choice for aerobic activity, especially if you're just starting out. It's inexpensive, simple, and carries a low risk of injury, but it can have a big impact on your health. Although walking is something you've likely been doing since you were a toddler, it's a good idea to brush up on proper techniques for fitness walking (see "Body Posture").

Begin by walking slowly to warm up, then increase your speed to a pace that raises your heart rate but still allows you to speak and breathe easily. When you have had enough, cool down by walking

NEW FINDING

Set Challenging but Achievable Goals

While striving to reach a goal is important, setting that bar too high can sabotage your effort, according to a new study from the Barcelona (Spain) Institute for Global Health. Researchers recruited 20 inactive overweight adults and sent them individualized daily step goals via a cell phone app. The goals ranged, at random, from the same number at baseline to more than twice as many. One day that might be 5,000 steps and the next perhaps 13,000. After 80 days, the researchers compared daily goals and overall activity levels. They found that people did walk more when their goals were higher, but most did not meet the highest step-count goals, sometimes walking even less than on the lower step-count days. The researchers found that goals that were just slightly out of reach were the ones that kept people motivated and moving. They concluded that goals should be challenging and achievable but also dynamic. For example, once a goal is consistently reached, they recommend increasing effort by 10 percent. Goals should be updated weekly, based on performance.

Health Psychology, January 2021

at a slower pace. Start at a distance and speed that are comfortable for you, then add five minutes a week until you are at your walking goal. It's important to set achievable goals, not too high and not too low is the best way to go, according to recent research (see "Set Challenging but Achievable Goals").

To step it up a notch, increase your intensity by adding hill or stair walking, wearing a weighted vest, and/or by increasing your speed. Nordic walking

Body Posture

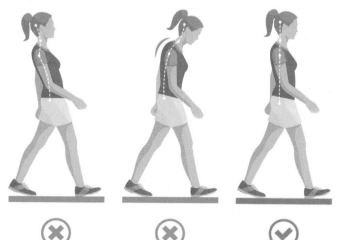

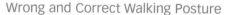

Wrong and Correct Walking Posture

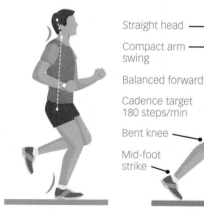

Straight head
Compact arm swing
Balanced forward
Cadence target 180 steps/min
Bent knee
Mid-foot strike

Wrong and Correct Running Posture

Whether you walk or run, good posture is important to ensure you get the most benefit out of your activity and, most importantly, don't hurt yourself. Maintain good posture and move with a comfortable stride. If you find that the activity increases or causes pain, consult with your physician and/or a personal trainer.

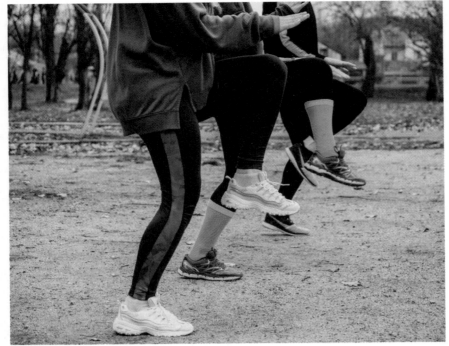
© Irinayeryomina | Dreamstime

High-intensity training doesn't have to be difficult. It simply must include a workout that raises your heart rate to 80 to 95 percent of its maximum heart rate.

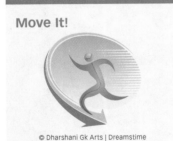
© Dharshani Gk Arts | Dreamstime

Move It!

Don't Walk Alone

Walking alone can be boring, but a furry friend with you can make everything more fun! Even if you don't own a pet, you may be able to volunteer at a rescue shelter and help walk homeless dogs (and maybe cats!). You'll be helping yourself, the animal, and the shelter—a win for all!

with poles adds the bonus of arm work; it's kind of like cross-country skiing on dry land that can be done in all seasons.

Strength Training

Performing muscle-strengthening activities at least two days a week helps preserve muscle and keep bones strong as you age. Also known as strength training or resistance training, this form of physical activity exercises a muscle or muscle group against external resistance. Resistance training slows down the loss of muscle mass and strength that occurs with age and helps keep bones strong.

Working hard against resistance—weights, stretchy resistance bands, or your own body weight—builds strength. Some of the benefits of regularly engaging in resistance exercise include:

- preserving or increasing muscle mass typically lost as you age
- maintaining your ability to perform activities of daily living in advanced age
- lowering body fat
- strengthening connective tissue around the muscle to prevent injury

- strengthening bones to help prevent osteoporosis
- decreasing blood pressure
- raising good (HDL) cholesterol levels

Muscle-strengthening exercises include push-ups, pull-ups, sit-ups, arm circles, lifting weights (free weights), using strength-training machines, working with resistance bands, and even climbing stairs, carrying heavy loads, and heavy gardening. Anything that provides something for your muscles to push or pull (weight resistance) can be used to increase muscle strength. Machine-based exercises are regarded as the safest form of resistance exercise for beginners.

Target each of the major muscle groups (legs, hips, chest, back, abdomen, shoulders, and arms) two to three times a week. The key is to perform each muscle-strengthening exercise until it would be difficult to perform the movement again without help. Do not exercise the same muscle groups on two consecutive days, however. After resistance exercise, muscles need recovery time, as your body starts to repair and replace damaged muscle fibers, forming new strands of muscle protein that result in stronger muscle tissue and, in some cases (particularly in younger individuals and men), bigger muscles.

A repetition, or "rep," is the number of times you perform a complete movement of a given exercise, such as a bicep curl. A "set" is a group of reps. If you do 10 bicep curls (10 reps), rest, and do 10 more, you have done two sets of 10 reps.

The development of muscle strength and endurance is progressive over time. When what you're doing becomes easy, add more repetitions. When you can do three sets of 10 to 15 reps easily, it is time to increase the weight or resistance you are using. Progressively overloading muscles is key to building strength. Rest one to three minutes between sets and between different exercises to keep your muscles from becoming overly tired.

Power Training

Muscle power—the combination of strength and speed that determines how quickly your muscles can produce a desired movement—may be even more important than muscle strength for preventing physical disability as you age. It's muscle power that gets you across a street before the light changes, allows you to hit the brakes quickly when another driver cuts you off, and helps you react swiftly when you trip so you don't fall.

A decline in muscle power has been shown to start earlier in the aging process and progress more quickly than loss of muscle strength. Researchers have found that a person's muscle power is a better predictor of their functional ability than their muscle strength. Given that lack of time is the No. 1 excuse for not exercising, researchers at the University of Texas at Austin wanted to see how much could be gained in training periods as short as 15 minutes. The short answer was quite a bit (see "Power Cycling Increases Muscle Mass and Power").

While strength-training exercises are traditionally performed relatively slowly, power training often involves doing the same exercises but contracting the muscles as quickly as possible (for example, bending your arms quickly in a bicep curl and straightening them more slowly, or rising from a chair as quickly as you can then gently sitting back down). Research has found high-velocity power training is safe and effective, even for frail elderly exercisers.

In a study of 45 older adults with self-reported mobility limitations, 12 weeks of high-velocity training improved muscle power approximately twice as much as a traditional strength-training program.

Power Cycling Increases Muscle Mass and Power

Previous research has shown that training at fast velocities results in superior muscle gain of fast-twitch muscle fibers compared to slow velocity training and greater improvements in maximal neuromuscular power. Researchers from the Human Performance Laboratory, Department of Kinesiology and Health Education at the University of Texas at Austin, wanted to know if very short intervals could result in meaningful gains. So, they recruited men and women to investigate the effectiveness of maximal power-cycling training using an inertial load cycle ergometer (a stationary bike with a weighted flywheel, such as those found in group cycling classes). The participants were 39 men and women between the ages of 50 and 68 with a body mass index of less than 30. They were free of overt heart disease, hypertension, or knee/hip joint problems. They were not engaged in systematic physical training.

Over the course of eight weeks, participants performed 15 minutes of interval training three times per week. Each session included repeated four-second sprints (with rest between) done at the person's maximum ability. Rest periods were progressively shortened from 56 seconds to 26 seconds during the eight-week period. At the end of the study, researchers reported that all participants showed significant improvements, especially in muscle power (about 12 percent), which is most relevant to functional tasks, according to the researchers. Function was tested by measuring how quickly participants could rise from a chair unassisted and timed walking speed. Both those tasks improved by the end of the eight-week study.

Medicine & Science in Sports and Exercise, June 2020

Other research shows that high-velocity resistance training also results in greater improvement in physical functioning in older adults, which is the key to remaining active and independent.

Fast-paced resistance exercise is the most-discussed form of power exercise, but research also has found benefits to stair-walking programs and the wearing of a weighted vest while performing certain basic activities. It's not necessary to use heavy weights or high resistance to increase your muscle power, although using heavier weights will lead to a greater increase in strength and endurance (see "Resistance Exercises").

All Movement Matters

Even if you don't reach the 150- to 300-minute weekly exercise target range,

Resistance Exercises

- calisthenics
- carrying heavy loads (including groceries)
- circuit training
- climbing stairs
- gardening (digging and lifting)
- lifting free weights
- Pilates
- some tai chi exercises
- some yoga exercises
- using weight machines
- using a medicine ball (weighted ball)
- working with resistance bands

Core Strength

Core muscles help you stand, bend, twist, reach, stoop, and turn. These are the muscles that surround your torso like a corset. They include your abdominals, back, shoulders, and hip muscles. When these muscles are strong, they help you stand up straight (rather than hunching over), and they promote good posture and balance, helping prevent falls. A strong core also helps reduce the likelihood of injuring your lower back.

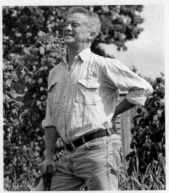
© Ian Allenden | Dreamstime

Lower-back pain may indicate a weak core.

When core muscles are weak, not only is physical activity more difficult, but eventually daily activities, such as getting dressed, carrying groceries, or vacuuming, can become a challenge. Signs of a weak core include poor posture, lower back pain, and muscle weakness in your arms and legs.

Clues you may have poor posture include a head that's commonly thrust forward, slouching, rounded shoulders, and excessive arching of your lower back with your stomach protruding. Sneak a peek at yourself in the mirror and see what your normal position is. While it can be scary, you'll get a reality check. Core exercises are especially valuable in improving posture.

Core muscles can and should be used during all activities. When the core is strong, it automatically supports what you are doing. Pilates, in particular, is designed to strengthen the core by challenging the muscles during a wide variety of movements. In short, to engage your core, pull in your muscles like you're trying to zip up a tight pair of jeans.

simply replacing sedentary behavior—like sitting at a desk, watching television, or reading—with light-intensity physical activity reduces the risk for premature death from any cause. It also has been found to reduce the risk of developing or dying from cardiovascular disease and decrease the risk for diabetes.

Perhaps a combination of mind-body exercise would fit better with your interest. Mind-body exercises have significant health benefits and are excellent low-impact ways to improve strength, flexibility, and balance. These exercise programs, which relax the mind while strengthening the body, continue to grow in popularity (see "Mind-Body Methods: Yoga, Tai Chi, Pilates").

If you're concerned that you don't have time for any exercise, data shows that there is no required duration of exercise sessions needed to achieve benefits. Any episodes of moderate-to-vigorous activity of any length can be added together to reach a daily total. And, if you are already achieving the physical activity target range, increasing your activity even further will enhance the substantial benefits you are already receiving from activity (see "Targeted Strength-Training Regimens by Goal").

Injury Prevention

Increase your level of physical activity slowly and choose workouts that are appropriate for any health conditions you may have. "No pain, no gain" has been proven wrong. If an activity hurts, stop doing it right away. Talk to your doctor before you begin any new exercise, especially if you have pain, tightness, or (Continued on page 20

Targeted Strength-Training Regimens by Goal

For Beginner to Intermediate Level: Doing any weight-bearing or resistance exercise is good for you. If you'd like to get more serious about lifting weights, this chart can help. Start by thinking about your goal: Do you want to be stronger? More powerful? Increase your endurance? How much weight you lift (load), how many times you perform an exercise (volume), how long you rest between sets (rest period), and how often you perform strength-training exercises (frequency) all depend on your goal.

GOAL ▶	MUSCLE STRENGTH: To increase the amount of weight you can lift.	POWER: To perform actions more quickly.	MUSCULAR ENDURANCE: To be able to perform activity longer.
load	Move heavier loads. Take your time.	Move moderately heavy loads at an intermediate velocity.	Choose a load that you can move many times before exhaustion.
volume	**Sets:** 1–3 **Reps:** 8–12	**Sets:** 1–3 **Reps:** 3–6	**Sets:** 2–4 **Reps:** 10–25
rest period (between sets)	**Lighter:** 1–2 minutes **Heavier:** 2–3 minutes	30 seconds to 1 minute	30 seconds to 1 minute
frequency	**Beginner:** Entire body 2–3 times per week. Include legs, hips, chest, back, abdomen, shoulders, and arms. **Intermediate:** 3 days per week if using total-body workouts; 4 days if using an upper/lower body split routine (training each major muscle group twice a week).		

Mind-Body Methods: Yoga, Tai Chi, Pilates

Mind-body exercise programs relax the mind while strengthening the body. Their popularity grows each year. You can choose to practice with or without a spiritual component designed to help users increase mindfulness or gain a deeper level of consciousness. There is no right or wrong choice. A 2020 study published in *Holistic Nurse Practice* that included 3,438 adults reported that yoga, tai chi, and qigong were effective in reducing low back pain, depression, and anxiety, and improving physical function.

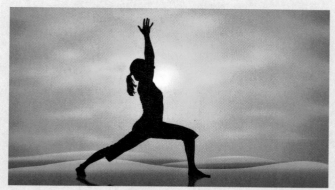

© Sandesh Patil | Dreamstime

Yoga

Yoga can be gentle and meditative or vigorous. A good instructor will demonstrate how each pose can be modified to fit your level of flexibility, balance, and conditioning, and most classes offer props like foam blocks, straps, and blankets to help you stay safe and comfortable in various positions. With its focus on postures and breathing, regular yoga practice may lower the risk for heart disease, with significant positive impacts on body weight, blood pressure, cholesterol, and triglycerides. Yoga, like aerobic exercise, has been linked to a decrease in depression. It also shows promise for managing arthritis, reducing stress, and improving sleep quality. A small trial, published in *Complementary Therapies in Clinical Practice* (2018), found that people with chronic pain and illnesses who practiced yoga over an eight-week period reported significantly less pain, better balance, increased upper and lower body strength, and a higher quality of life compared to those who did not practice yoga.

Tai Chi

This ancient Chinese mind-body practice combines martial arts with meditation. It is a series of slow movements that are performed with attention to posture and breathing and an awareness of the interplay between force and relaxation. Tai Chi Easy is a specific program designed to be accessible to beginners.

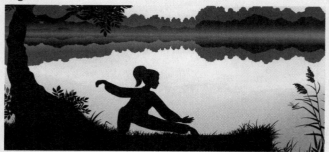

© Elokuu | Dreamstime

Tai chi is said to improve physical, mental, and spiritual well-being. Research indicates it also shows promise for reduction of stress, anxiety, and depression. It's also been reported to be as good as physical therapy for reducing osteoarthritis pain and may be helpful for patients suffering with fibromyalgia. A study published in *JAMA Internal Medicine* reported that tai chi was effective for reducing fall risk by 31 percent in the group of 670 study participants ages 70 and older.

Pilates

Pilates is a non-impact exercise program designed to strengthen your core muscles while simultaneously developing flexibility, balance, control, coordination, and proprioception (awareness of where you are in space). It quickly became popular with dancers and other athletes to help them recover from injuries and improve performance.

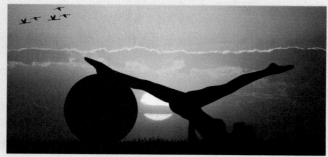

© Adrenalinapura | Dreamstime

In Pilates, quality is much more important than quantity. The twisting, stretching, pushing, pulling, and rolling exercises are either done on the floor in mat classes or on specialized spring-based machines. The machines provide both resistance and assistance, which helps you learn the key principles more quickly and deeply. This full-body exercise modality is an excellent choice for post rehab and to enhance any activity, be it golf, tennis, or picking up the grandkids.

Pilates is best started on equipment as a one-on-one training experience with a certified Pilates instructor who has at least 500 hours of education. Because it requires focused, precise, and controlled movements that actively stretch and strengthen the body at the same time, Pilates has become an increasingly popular exercise program within physical therapy centers. A study reported in *Musculoskeletal Care* found that a 12-week individualized Pilates program significantly reduced pain in those with chronic low back pain, osteoarthritis, and postsurgical conditions. Many study participants reported feeling surprised at how much Pilates "turned back the clock" as they felt they were still improving their fitness, despite advancing age.

(Continued from page 18)

pressure in your chest during normal activity; if you often experience dizziness or lightheadedness; if you have high blood pressure, pain, stiffness, or swelling that limits activity; or if you feel unsteady or are prone to falls.

Choosing the right workout for your needs or physical limitations and learning the proper technique for performing each exercise can keep you from hurting yourself. Varying your workouts so you

Warm Up, Cool Down

Warming up helps gradually increase your heart rate and breathing, improving the delivery of oxygen and fuel to working muscles. And it only takes five to 10 minutes. It warms your muscles so they're ready to work, which reduces the risk of injury and muscle soreness after exercise.

Avoid static stretches—stretching to a challenging but comfortable position and holding it for several seconds—during the warm-up. Save these for the cool down when muscles are warm. A few ideas of how to warm up include:

- Walk around or march in place while swinging your arms, along with some knee lifts and small kicks.
- Walk up and down stairs a few times.
- Dance around your living room to a couple of songs.
- Mimic some of the same movements you'll be doing during the actual exercise, but at a slower pace and lower intensity. For example: Warm up for a walk by walking slowly at first, then gradually increase your pace.
- If you're going to play tennis, hit some easy groundstrokes from the middle of the court. Or, if you are going to play a round of golf, warm up by taking some easy swings on the driving range.

In addition, remember to take about five to 10 minutes at the end of your workout to cool down. It's like the warm-up but in reverse and can include some flexibility stretches and relaxation breathing. Stretching at the end of your cool down may help increase your range of motion in future exercise. Stretch the same muscles you worked during your exercise session.

Cooling down at the end of your exercise session helps you gradually decrease your body temperature, heart rate, and breathing, as well as reduce the risk of dizziness associated with abruptly stopping exercise. Keeping your arm and leg muscles moving during the cool down helps prevent blood from pooling in your hands and feet and can help reduce muscle stiffness after your session.

aren't stressing the same muscle groups every time is important as well.

The main risk is that your muscles may be sore in the first few weeks of starting an exercise program. Although you likely won't be able to avoid this, and it's important to challenge yourself, one of the best ways to reduce muscle soreness is to gradually progress in your exercise program rather than trying to do too much at the start. Muscle soreness generally resolves by itself within a few days.

Warming up and cooling down also can help prevent injury. Warming up before exercise helps provide a safe transition to moving your body, and cooling down at the end of a session supports your body's recovery after exercise (see "Warm Up, Cool Down").

While a mix of aerobic and strength-training exercise is ideal—and mind-body and power training are valuable—any activity, at any level, is better than none. Remember that the benefits of exercise begin to accrue after just one session.

According to the Physical Activity Guidelines for Americans Advisory Committee, just one bout of moderate-to-vigorous physical activity will reduce blood pressure, boost insulin sensitivity, enhance sleep, reduce anxiety symptoms, and perk up cognition on the day that it is performed.

Being active on a regular basis makes these improvements even larger. The reduction in disease risk and improved physical function can be seen within days to weeks after adopting a new physical-activity routine. So, get up and get yourself moving!

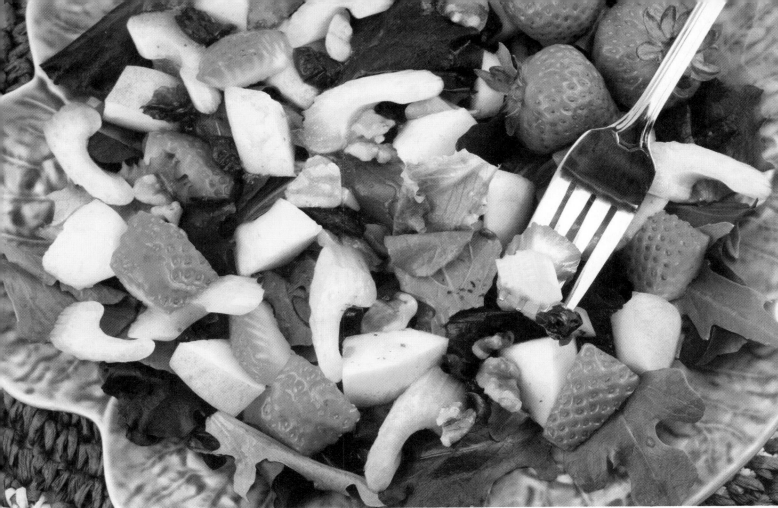

© Davisflowerlady | Dreamstime

3 Key Nutrients for Healthy Aging

Have you ever opened the refrigerator when you weren't super hungry just looking for something to snack on? Many people eat when just mildly hungry, and there's nothing particularly wrong with that as long as you're choosing foods that benefit your health. Snacking on the right foods (low in calories, high in nutrition) can help quell hunger pangs and provide you with optimum nutrients to sustain energy.

When snacking, select whole foods with little processing, and look for sources of healthy mono- and polyunsaturated fats, whole grains, and fiber. For example, enjoy a cheese stick with an apple or small bunch of grapes, nibble on a banana with a light smear of nut butter, or a eat a tuna snack pack with whole grain crackers. And consider the benefits of this wonderful snack—eating a few walnuts daily can help keep your heart happy (see "Walnuts May Reduce Heart Disease").

A healthy salad filled with strawberries, apples, celery, and low-sugar dried cranberries, topped with walnuts on a bed of mixed spring lettuce with raspberry vinaigrette dressing. Sounds great, doesn't it?

NEW FINDING

Walnuts May Reduce Heart Disease

Including a few walnuts in your daily eating plan may ward off heart disease. The delicious nuts may have anti-inflammatory properties that are linked with a lower risk for cardiovascular disease, according to a study published in the *Journal of American Cardiology.* The researchers divided 634 healthy older adults (ages 63 to 94) into two groups. The first group consumed 1 to 2 ounces (about 14 to 28 walnut halves) each day for two years. The second group continued with their usual day without walnuts. At the end of the study, participants who ate walnuts had lower amounts of six inflammatory markers that are linked to heart disease, compared to those who didn't consume walnuts daily. Chronic inflammation is a critical factor in the development and progression of atherosclerosis, which is the buildup of plaque or "hardening" of the arteries, the principal cause of heart attacks and stroke. The research was part of the Walnuts and Healthy Aging Study, the largest, longest trial exploring the benefits of daily walnut consumption.

Journal of American Cardiology, Nov. 10, 2020

Vitamin D May Reduce COVID-19 Risk

Research led from the School of Public Health, Tulane University, New Orleans, investigated the relationship between vitamin D and the risk of coronavirus disease 2019 (COVID-19) infection. Previous studies have reported that vitamin D supplementation may lower the risk of acute respiratory tract infection, and evidence during the pandemic suggested that vitamin D insufficiency is related to a higher risk of severe COVID-19 infection. The study data came from the UK Biobank, a population cohort study that included participants ages 37 to 73. For the study, researchers looked at data from 8,297 adults, their use of vitamin D supplements, and records of their COVID-19 test results. Researchers found that habitual use of vitamin D supplements was associated with a lower risk of COVID-19 infection, independent of lifestyle, socioeconomic status, and prevalent chronic diseases. Use of the supplement was associated with a 34 percent lower risk of COVID-19 infection. According to the researchers, further study is needed to verify the results.

American Journal of Clinical Nutrition, Jan. 29, 2021

Making smart dietary decisions becomes ever more important as we age because the body becomes less tolerant of junk food and less efficient at absorbing key nutrients. A few key nutrients are especially valuable for healthy aging:

- **Protein** is vital for just about everything the body does including building, maintaining, and repairing muscles, bones, and skin; as well helping to make enzymes, hormones, and neurotransmitters. Good sources of protein include animal-based foods (e.g., chicken, fish, eggs, milk) and plant-based protein sources such as seeds (e.g., pumpkin, hemp), almonds, oats, beans, and tofu.

- **Vitamin D** promotes the absorption of calcium and plays a role in immune function, brain health, insulin regulation and other vital processes. It's called the sunshine vitamin because the skin makes vitamin D when exposed to sunlight, but this ability declines with age. Fatty fish and fish oil are good sources of vitamin D, as are fortified foods such as dairy and alternative milks, orange juice, and breakfast cereals. Its immune-boosting ability was especially relevant regarding COVID-19 (see "Vitamin D May Reduce COVID-19 Risk").

- **Fiber** is lacking in most people's diets. It is great for reducing cholesterol, aiding digestion and bowel movements, and assisting in weight loss by increasing the feeling of fullness. Whole fruits and veggies are excellent sources, especially with the skin on, when possible. Be sure to drink more fluids when you increase fiber to help keep waste moving along through the intestines.

- **Calcium** is essential for lowering blood pressure, preventing osteoporosis, and preserving bone health. For maximum absorption of calcium, it can be helpful to spread out intake throughout the day. Good sources include hard cheeses, nuts, seeds, yogurt, and veggies such as kale, broccoli, and watercress.

- **Vitamin B_{12}** becomes more difficult to extract from foods as we age. It's needed for proper blood cell formation and neurological function. A vitamin B_{12} deficiency can mimic symptoms of dementia. If that's the case, replenishing B_{12} can reverse cognitive problems. Find B_{12} in fish, eggs, poultry, and fortified sources such as breakfast cereal, not a supplement pill.

Obviously, some foods contain many of these nutrients, making it easy to put together nutrient-rich snacks and meals. For example, raspberries with nuts and seeds sprinkled on yogurt check off virtually all the above. Creative combinations can help inspire you when it comes to meal prep. The recipes at the end of this report are an example of how delicious and easy healthy eating can be.

Switch to Healthy

We each have our own dietary pattern—what we eat and drink—and making that a *healthy* dietary pattern means focusing on what you *can* eat instead of what you can't. Healthy dietary patterns ensure you get everything you need so you function optimally. And nutritious foods help energize the body and keep the mind clear and sharp.

The best diet is a proportion-appropriate eating plan that provides all the nutrients you need to live well, fight disease, be active, and maintain a healthy weight. The current recommendations and tools can make it easier for you to discover and build your ideal eating pattern.

Make Every Bite Count

Every five years, the U.S. Department of Health and Human Services and the U.S. Department of Agriculture (USDA) jointly publish a report with nutritional and dietary information and guidelines. This report, called *the Dietary Guidelines for Americans*, is required to be based on the latest scientific and medical knowledge. While previous editions focused primarily on individual dietary components, such as food groups and nutrients, the 2020–2025 *Dietary Guidelines for Americans* is the first to time the experts provided guidance by stage of life, from birth to older adulthood, including pregnancy and lactation. The *Guidelines* continue to focuses on the combination of foods and beverages that make up an individual's whole diet over time and not single foods or eating occasions in isolation. Research shows that the ongoing pattern of an individual's eating habits has the greatest impact on their health (see "Dietary Guidelines for Americans").

The Importance of Portions

To make it easier to figure out if you are eating the right foods in the right proportions for optimal health, use the USDA's MyPlate (see "MyPlate"), a visual guideline that serves as a reminder of what constitutes a healthy dietary pattern. MyPlate shows half of a nine-inch plate covered with fruits and vegetables, with less than a quarter reserved for protein and slightly more than a quarter for grains. In 2021, a new app was introduced to help people simplify food planning. Pick goals based on your needs, see real time progress, take quizzes, find recipes, join challenges and more. Get the details here: tinyurl.com/myplateapp.

Fruits and Veggies

It's no surprise that fruits and vegetables make up one-half of the MyPlate plate. It is recommended that women and men over 19 years old aim for 1½ to 2 cups of fruit a day and 2½ to 3 cups of vegetables a day, respectively.

Fruits and vegetables are generally low in fat, sodium, and calories, and provide many essential nutrients that tend to be lacking in the American diet, including blood-pressure-lowering potassium, cholesterol-lowering fiber, wound-healing vitamin C, and vitamin A, which keeps eyes and skin healthy and helps protect against infections.

A colorful plate is beautiful, delicious, keeps meals interesting, and ensures you get a variety of phytochemicals and other nutrients. Buy fresh produce in season for the best flavor and lowest price, but stock up on frozen fruits and vegetables, which are often even more

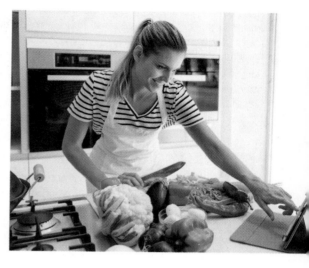

© Nenitorx | Dreamstime

Healthy recipes are plentiful on the internet, and we share some in the back of this Special Health Report, too.

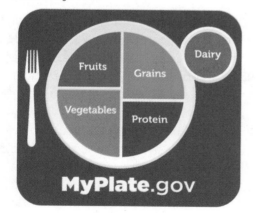

USDA MyPlate

The USDA's MyPlate graphic is based on recommendations from the *Dietary Guidelines for Americans*.

Dietary Guidelines for Americans

EAT MORE...	AND LESS...
• **vegetables of all types:** dark green; red and orange; beans, peas, and lentils; starchy; and other vegetables • **fruits,** especially whole fruit • **grains,** at least half of which are whole grain • **dairy,** including fat-free or low-fat milk, yogurt, and cheese, and/or lactose-free versions and fortified soy beverages and yogurt as alternatives • **protein foods,** including lean meats, poultry, and eggs; seafood; beans, peas, and lentils; and nuts, seeds, and soy products • **oils,** including vegetable oils and oils in food, such as seafood and nuts	• **added sugars:** Less than 10 percent of calories per day starting at age 2. Avoid foods and beverages with added sugars for those younger than age 2. • **saturated fat:** Less than 10 percent of calories per day starting at age 2. • **sodium:** Less than 2,300 milligrams per day—and even less for children younger than age 14. • **alcoholic beverages:** Adults of legal drinking age can choose not to drink, or to drink in moderation by limiting intake to 2 drinks or less in a day for men and 1 drink or less in a day for women, when alcohol is consumed. Drinking less is better for health than drinking more. There are some adults who should not drink alcohol, such as women who are pregnant.

Convenient, Frozen, and Nutrient-Rich

Fresh produce that needs to travel to grocery stores is often picked early, so it never reaches its full nutrient potential, and some nutrient levels go down over time as the produce is shipped and then sits, waiting to be purchased. On the other hand, fruits and vegetables that are to be frozen usually fully ripen on the plant and are frozen and packaged within hours of harvest, preserving peak flavor and nutritional value.

The downside, however, is the added sodium, saturated fat, and sugar in some products. Read labels! Look for fruits that have no added sugar. Skip frozen vegetables with fat- or sodium-laden sauces.

Source: Produce for Better Health Foundation

Understanding One-Ounce Equivalents

It is recommended that adults consume five to seven servings (called ounce-equivalents) of grains a day, depending on their calorie needs. Below are a few examples of what counts as a serving of grains.

Aim to make at least half of your grain servings whole-grain foods. Look for the Whole Grains Stamp on packaged foods to find out how many grams of whole grains are in the serving size listed on the label. Aim for at least 48 grams of whole grains a day.

GRAINS	ONE-OUNCE EQUIVALENT
bagels	• 1 mini bagel
breads	• 1 regular slice
bulgur	• ½ cup cooked
crackers	• 5 whole-wheat crackers • 2 rye crispbreads • 7 square or round crackers
English muffins	• ½ muffin
oatmeal	• ½ cup cooked • 1 packet instant • ⅓ cup dry
popcorn	• 3 cups, popped
pasta or rice	• ½ cup cooked • 1 ounce uncooked
ready-to-eat breakfast cereals	• 1 cup, flakes or rounds • 1¼ cups puffed
tortilla	• 1 corn or flour tortilla (6 in. diameter)

Source: ChooseMyPlate.gov

nutritious than fresh and more economical (see "Convenient, Frozen, and Nutrient-Rich"). Enjoying these delicious plants doesn't just provide you with better health now; eating a variety of produce may pay off in years to come. Studies show people who eat the highest concentration of fruits and vegetables score better on cognitive tests.

Canned vegetables can be a good choice as well, but watch out for added sodium. Cans labeled "reduced sodium," "low sodium," or "no salt added" are a better choice, even if you add a little salt at home. Some people feel that without salt foods taste bland.

Chili peppers—which come in a variety of heat indexes (Scoville Heat Units) range from mild (paprika, pepperoncini) to medium (poblano, jalapeno) to scorching (habanero, Carolina reaper)—add not only heat, but unique spicy flavor profiles. According to a 2019 study from Italy, published in the *Journal of the American College of Cardiology*, people who eat chili peppers on a regular basis lower their risk of dying from heart disease by as much as 30 percent. Capsaicin is the key compound that makes the pepper hot, and it may be responsible for quelling inflammation as well as other harmful processes involved in the formation of arterial plaque. Researchers also theorize that people who use hot chili peppers may use fewer other ingredients, such as butter and salt, that may be heart-harming.

Fruit is easy to add to breakfast, throw in a bag for a snack or lunch side, or toss into salads, but it's also delicious paired with meat dishes, such as chicken with apricots or pineapple on kabobs. Baked apples, poached pears, and fruit salad also make a satisfyingly sweet dessert.

Upping your veggie intake is not difficult. Main-dish salads make easy and versatile meals. Toss extra veggies into soups, stews, stir-fries, and casseroles. Top pizza with extra veggies. Add a side salad in place of an extra slice.

Protein Essentials

The Protein Foods Group includes all foods made from meat, poultry, seafood, beans, peas, eggs, processed soy products, nuts, and seeds. Protein makes up about one-quarter of the MyPlate plate, and nutritionists recommend that men and women over 19 years old consume 5½- to 6½-ounce equivalents of protein a day (see "Understanding One-Ounce Equivalents").

Protein provides the building blocks for bone, muscle, cartilage, skin, and blood, as well as enzymes, hormones, and vitamins. Plant and animal protein sources also supply energy-producing B vitamins, antioxidant vitamin E, oxygen-carrying iron, zinc for your immune system, and magnesium to help build strong bones and release energy from muscles when needed.

Despite protein's role as a building block for muscle, it can't reverse the effects of aging. A 2018 study from the Institute of Medicine, which included 92 men ages 65 and older, found that simply eating extra protein above the current recommended daily allowance (RDA) does not reverse the muscle loss that comes with aging.

Ideal Protein. The type of protein you choose matters. Along with protein, you may be consuming high levels of heart-harming saturated fat (from foods like red meat, poultry skin, and full-fat dairy) and sodium (from cured meats like ham), or cancer-causing nitrates from processed meats (sausage, bacon, beef jerky). Likewise, you could get beneficial omega-3 fatty acids (from fish) or fiber and antioxidants (from legumes).

Diets that are high in saturated fats, from foods like red meat and full-fat dairy, raise LDL ("bad") cholesterol levels in the blood and increase the risk for coronary heart disease. Choose low-fat dairy products and lean meat, and remove the skin from poultry to cut down on your saturated fat intake. Lean cuts of beef include round steaks and roasts, top loin, top sirloin, and chuck shoulder and arm roasts. Choose ground beef that is at least 92 percent lean. Pork loin, tenderloin, center loin, and ham are the leanest cuts of pork.

Aim to consume 8 ounces of seafood a week to help prevent heart disease. All seafood is good, but salmon, trout, sardines, anchovies, herring, Pacific oysters, and Atlantic and Pacific mackerel are particularly high in heart-healthy omega-3 fatty acids. While there has been some concern about high mercury levels in fish, the health benefits from consuming seafood outweigh any health risk from mercury. DHA is a type of omega-3 fatty acid found in fish that is particularly helpful to brain health (see "Fish and Brain Health").

Beans and peas are classified as both vegetables and protein sources. These mature legumes (such as chickpeas, kidney beans, pinto beans, black beans, black-eyed peas, split peas, and lentils) are great sources of fiber and nutrients such as potassium and folate. They are also excellent sources of plant protein and provide you with iron and zinc, two nutrients that are found in meats, poultry, and fish.

Although they make great vegetarian alternatives to meat, legumes are an excellent addition to any diet. (Green peas, green lima beans, and green string beans are not good protein sources and are not included in this group.) Toss beans on salads, into soups, stews, and chili; use hummus or another bean purée as a sandwich spread or dip; or spice them up and serve over grain.

Vary your protein sources to get the most from this part of your meal. Seafood, beans, and soy products are a great break from meats (beef, veal, lamb, pork, and chicken). Enjoy them as a main dish or side dish frequently. Eating nuts and seeds as part of a balanced dietary pattern is associated with a reduced risk of heart disease, but choose unsalted varieties to keep sodium intake down, and eat them in small portions to avoid excess calories (see "Portioning Protein Sources" on the following page).

People tend to eat most of their protein at the evening meal, with little protein at breakfast. Research suggests that consuming protein at breakfast, lunch, and dinner may better support your ability to maintain muscle mass as you age.

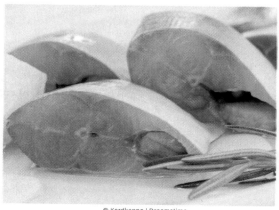
© Kerdkanno | Dreamstime

The acronym SMASH stands for salmon, mackerel (pictured), anchovies, sardines, and herring, all of which are low in mercury and high in omega-3s.

NEW FINDING

Fish and Brain Health

Older women who eat more than one to two servings a week of baked or broiled fish or shellfish may consume enough omega-3 fatty acids to counteract the effects of air pollution on the brain, according to a study funded by the National Institutes of Health. Researchers found that among older women who lived in areas with high levels of air pollution, those who had the lowest levels of omega-3 fatty acids in their blood had more brain shrinkage than women who had the highest levels. The study included 1,315 Caucasian women, average age 70, who did not have dementia at the start of the study. They completed questionnaires about diet, physical activity, and medical history. Researchers used the women's home addresses to determine their exposure to air pollution. Study participants underwent brain scans and blood tests to determine the amount of omega-3 fatty acids in their blood. Women who had the highest levels of omega-3 fatty acids in the blood had greater volumes of white matter in the brain than those with the lowest levels. They also had greater volumes of the hippocampus, an area of the brain that plays a major role in learning and memory.
Neurology, July 15, 2020

Portioning Protein Sources

Aim for 5½- to 6½-ounce equivalents of protein a day. Both animal- and plant-based foods supply protein. Be sure to include a plant or animal protein source at every meal. When eating animal proteins, opt for lean and low-fat products. Most plant proteins are low in one or more essential amino acids; eat a variety of plant foods to help provide all the amino acids your body needs.

PROTEIN	OUNCE-EQUIVALENT
beans (baked, refried, black, kidney, pinto, white, etc.)	¼ cup
egg	1 large egg; 2 egg whites
Falafel	1 patty (2¼ inch)
hummus	2 tablespoons
meats (lean beef, lean pork or ham)	1 ounce
nut butter	1 tablespoon
nuts (12 almonds, 24 pistachios, 7 walnut halves)	½ ounce
peas (chickpeas, cowpeas, lentils, split peas)	¼ cup
poultry, skinless	1 ounce, 1 sandwich slice
quinoa, cooked*	½ cup
seafood (cooked fish or shellfish)	1 ounce
seeds (pumpkin, sunflower, squash, hulled and roasted)	½ ounce
soybeans, roasted	¼ cup
tempeh*	1 ounce
tofu*	¼ cup (about 2 ounces)

Source: ChooseMyPlate.gov. *A "complete protein" plant source that provides all essential amino acids.

Valuable Whole Grains

According to MyPlate, grains or grain-based foods should make up about a quarter of your meal. All adults should consume six to eight ounce-equivalents of grains a day, of which three to four are whole grains.

Whole grains have fiber, several B vitamins, and minerals like iron, magnesium, and immune-boosting selenium. Like fruits and vegetables, whole grains have powerful phytochemicals. Consuming whole grains may reduce your risk of heart disease, ease constipation, reduce inflammation, and aid in weight management.

When grains are refined—to turn whole wheat into white flour, or brown rice into white rice, for example—most of these nutrients (and their health benefits) are stripped away. Americans eat a lot of products made from refined wheat flour (white bread, pasta, baked goods), far exceeding recommended amounts of refined grains and falling short on dietary recommendations for consuming whole grains.

Scientists with the Jean Mayer USDA Human Nutrition Research Center on Aging at Tufts University studied the effects of whole grains in 2017 and found that eating them helped with weight loss. Women who ate a minimum of 3 ounces daily and men who consumed 4 ounces lost about 100 calories more per day compared to study participants who didn't eat grains.

Try to eat whole grains at least three times a day. If this seems like a lot, start by switching out one refined-grain food for a whole-grain version. For example, start the day with oatmeal or whole-grain cereal instead of refined choices at breakfast, use whole-grain bread at lunch, and serve whole grains as a side dish at dinner. For a powerful combination of healthful nutrients in just the balance nature intended, choose delicious whole grains of all kinds (such as wheat, barley, brown rice, quinoa, and oats).

Eating brown rice in place of white rice is one option, but consider trying other grains, too. Barley is a delicious choice and can be used in place of rice as a side dish and in many recipes, like soups, pilafs, and grain-based salads.

Quinoa is quick and easy to cook and versatile, and it's one of the rare plant sources of protein that contains all the essential amino acids. At snack time, you can swap in popcorn in place of pretzels or try eating whole-grain crackers instead of refined.

If you're eating processed foods, keep in mind that whole-grain options can still be high in added sugars and/or saturated fat. For example, whole-grain muffins, although better than their refined-grain counterparts, may contain a lot of sugar and/or saturated fat and should be eaten in moderation. And, while popcorn is a whole-grain food, sugar-coated or buttery popcorn isn't the optimal whole-grain choice (see "Cut the Sugar").

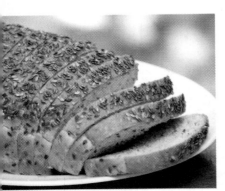

© Alfredo Angeles | Dreamstime

Once you've made the switch to nutritious, delicious, and satisfying baked goods made with whole grains, you'll never want to go back to refined grains.

Variety Is Vital

All the foods on your plate are a combination of nutrients: macronutrients (protein, carbohydrates, and fats) that provide calories for energy; micronutrients (vitamins and minerals) necessary for body functions; fiber for digestive health and to support a healthy gut microbiome; and powerful antioxidant and anti-inflammatory phytochemicals. A balanced dietary pattern ensures you get the nutrients and food components you need to stay healthy. Micronutrients are essential to everyone, but especially to those with chronic conditions, such as heart-failure patients. A 2018 study published in the *Journal of the American Heart Association* showed that a varied diet is necessary to prevent these individuals from having multiple micronutrient deficiencies and the resulting adverse health consequences.

Be Carb Wise

Carbohydrates are not necessarily bad. We should get 45 to 65 percent of our calories from carbs. Carbs are sugars or chains of sugars that serve as the primary fuel for the human body. We get carbs from health-promoting whole grains, fruits, vegetables, legumes, and dairy, but also from refined grain products, sweets, and sugary drinks that typically fall short on the vitamins, minerals, fiber, and phytochemicals found naturally in whole foods.

Whole-food carbs not only provide more of what your body needs for good health, they also tend to be gentler on blood-sugar levels than refined-carbohydrate and sugary foods. Once glucose is in your bloodstream, your pancreas releases insulin to help move the glucose into cells. Because whole foods are generally higher in fiber and move through your digestive tract

Cut the Sugar

Sugars found in the typical Western diet have been linked to high triglyceride levels, high cholesterol, high blood pressure, and weight gain. The average American consumes 15.4 teaspoons of added sugars every day, according to the American Heart Association.

The American Heart Association advises sugar intake at:

- **Women.** No more than 6 teaspoons (25 grams) a day
- **Men.** No more than 9 teaspoons (38 grams) a day

There are 4.2 grams of sugar in a teaspoon. For a quick way to picture how much sugar is in a serving of the foods you buy, find "sugars" and "added sugars" on the Nutrition Facts label and apply the following formula: _____ total grams of sugar divided by 4 = _____ approximate teaspoons of sugar.

Source: American Heart Association

If you concentrate on choosing good carbs, the sugary ones eventually won't be as appealing.

© VectorMine | Dreamstime

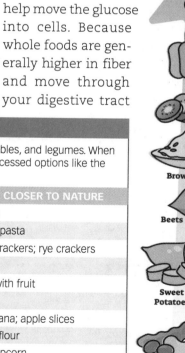

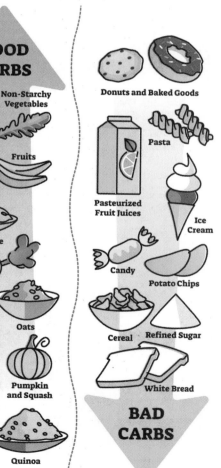

Not All Carbs Are Equal

Aim to get your carbs from whole grains, fruits, vegetables, and legumes. When choosing packaged foods, consider natural or less-processed options like the ones below.

HIGHLY PROCESSED	NATURAL OR CLOSER TO NATURE
instant, flavored oatmeal	steel-cut oats
white-flour pasta	whole-wheat pasta
refined-grain crackers	whole-grain crackers; rye crackers
fig cookie	dried figs
pudding	plain yogurt with fruit
orange drink	orange
grape jelly	smashed banana; apple slices
all-purpose flour	whole-wheat flour
pretzels	air-popped popcorn
potato chips	oven-roasted sweet potato slices
apple slices with caramel dip	apple slices with natural nut butter
white bread	whole-grain bread

more slowly, glucose from these foods is absorbed into your bloodstream more slowly and steadily. As a result, your body doesn't have to release as much insulin to take care of the glucose, so your blood sugar is stable, and you feel better. Avoiding big spikes in insulin followed by large drops in blood sugar can help keep your appetite in check, too.

When it comes to carbs, quality is key, not quantity. Instead of limiting carbs, choose whole-food "good carbs" like whole grains, beans, fruits, and vegetables over refined grains and sweets (see "Not All Carbs Are Equal").

Know Your Fats

Approximately 25 to 35 percent of your daily calories should come from fats. Since fats have 9 calories per gram (as opposed to protein and carbs, which have 4), it doesn't take a lot of fat to meet this recommendation. Dietary fats are necessary for the absorption of fat-soluble vitamins A, D, E, and K from foods. Fats also give foods a pleasant feel and carry flavor across our tongues, which is why low-fat ice cream doesn't feel or taste the same as full-fat ice cream. While the calorie density of fats can lead to weight gain, eating some dietary fat is necessary, and some kinds of fat are essential, since the body can't make them on its own.

All fats can be classified as either saturated or unsaturated. Saturated fats (found in animal products and tropical oils like palm and coconut) have been linked to an increased risk of cardiovascular disease, and all major medical organizations recommend limiting saturated fat intake to 10 percent or less of daily calories, which is about 22 grams of fat daily for a 2,000-calorie diet (see "Limiting Saturated Fat"). Most Americans currently get more than this recommended amount of saturated fat.

When unsaturated fats (whether mono- or polyunsaturated) replace saturated fats in the diet, the risk of cardiovascular disease goes down. Monounsaturated fats (found in most vegetable oils, nuts, seeds, and avocados) seem to raise HDL ("good") cholesterol and lower LDL ("bad") cholesterol and triglyceride levels in the blood. Polyunsaturated fats (in plant oils, fish, nuts, seeds, and soybeans) also can help reduce LDL cholesterol. This class of fats contains the two fatty acids your body can't make on its own: the essential fatty acids omega-3 and omega-6.

Eating patterns high in omega-3 fats have been shown to reduce inflammation and promote healing after exercise and may increase synthesis of new muscle.

Although fatty fish—like salmon, mackerel, herring, and trout—are by far the top source of the most potent omega-3 fats, you'll get smaller amounts of omega-3 fats in grass-fed beef (typically sold at farmers markets or health-food stores), walnuts, ground flaxseed, and chia seeds. Omega-6s, common in plant oils, are ubiquitous in the Western diet since they are used often in processed foods.

Since they are higher in calories than other macronutrients, all fats contribute more readily to unwanted weight gain (including inflammatory abdominal fat), regardless of whether they are classified as "good fat" or "bad fat" from a health perspective.

How Plants Protect

Special compounds in plants help protect them from disease and repair damage. When you eat plants (fruit, vegetables, whole grains, legumes, nuts, and

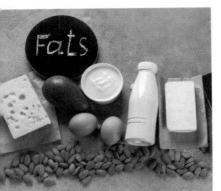

© Tatjana Baibakova | Dreamstime

Many people don't understand that fats contain more calories per gram than protein or carbohydrates.

Limiting Saturated Fat			
SOURCE/REFERENCE	Percent of total calories	Maximum daily saturated fat grams	
		2,000-calorie diet	1,800-calorie diet
Dietary Guidelines for Americans	10 percent	22	20
American Heart Association	7 percent	15.5	14
American Heart Association for people with high cholesterol	5–6 percent	11–13	10–12

seeds), those same compounds help protect your cells from disease and repair damage as well. Free radicals, which are compounds that have inflammatory cell- and tissue-damaging effects, form in your body from normal everyday body processes, such as metabolism. The metabolic activity of intense exercise also generates free radicals, but this is largely offset by the fact that exercise up-regulates the body's natural defenses against them as well. Eating plant foods helps fight these pro-aging compounds.

Plants contain compounds called phytochemicals (plant chemicals) that have powerful impacts on the human body. Some examples you may be familiar with are lycopene in tomatoes and watermelon (which reduces prostate cancer risk) and lutein in spinach and kiwi (to help prevent age-related blindness). Carotenoids, which make plants yellow, orange, and reddish, are beneficial to the cardiovascular system and may help reduce Alzheimer's disease (see "Carotenoids May Reduce Plaques and Tangles"). Plant-based foods also are good sources of a variety of antioxidants. These phytochemicals neutralize free radicals, helping to keep cells healthy and reduce systemic inflammation and the risk of diseases, like cancer and cardiovascular disease.

In addition, researchers have found the lack of carotenoids may weaken muscles (see "The Effect of Antioxidant Effect on Grip Strength and Gait Speed").

Although thousands of phytochemicals in foods have been identified, scientists suspect that many more exist. Because we don't know all of the many health-promoting phytochemicals in foods, consuming whole foods may be better than trying to increase your intake of a single specific nutrient with a dietary supplement. Food components act in concert to produce a symphony of beneficial effects, so isolating individual components into supplements could produce unsatisfactory or unexpected results.

Healthy Eating Made Easy

MyPlate is a simple guide to a balanced, varied, and portion-controlled dietary pattern, but there are other ways to approach healthy eating. The Mediterranean diet, the Dietary Approaches to Stop Hypertension (DASH) diet, and plant-based diets have all been extensively studied and found to provide major health benefits.

Mediterranean Diet

This diet refers to the traditional eating pattern of people in countries that surround the Mediterranean Sea (e.g., Italy, Greece, Turkey, Israel, and Morocco). A Mediterranean diet focuses on vegetables, fruits, whole grains, legumes, seafood, herbs, spices, nuts, and healthy fats, minimizing red meat and sweets. Wine (one five-ounce glass for women and two for men) can be enjoyed, if desired.

Olive trees are common in the Mediterranean, and olive oil—particularly extra virgin olive oil—is a key part of Mediterranean eating. The monounsaturated fats

NEW FINDING

Carotenoids May Reduce Plaques and Tangles

A long-term study, the Rush Memory and Aging Project, included 927 older individuals with no dementia at the start of the study. The volunteers filled out questionnaires about what they ate. Those with the highest intake of carotenoids were only half as likely to develop Alzheimer's disease (AD). Carotenoids are colorful compounds that give plants yellow, orange, and reddish hues. Lots of produce contains carotenoids, including pumpkin, squash, tomatoes, peas, kale, oranges, and cantaloupes. During the study, 508 people died and underwent autopsy. Those who consumed more carotenoids were less likely to have tangles and plaques, which are hallmarks of AD.
American Journal of Clinical Nutrition, January 2021

NEW FINDING

The Effect of Antioxidants on Grip Strength and Gait Speed

Sarcopenia, which is the age-related decline in muscle, can cause considerable problems in older adults and sets the stage not only for mobility impairments but also for cardiovascular disease. The causes are multifactorial and not fully understood. But evidence does show that a lack of exercise and an inadequate intake of vitamin D and dietary protein certainly play a role in sarcopenia. It's suspected that oxidative stress may also diminish function. Researchers included investigators from Harvard Medical School and the Jean Mayer USDA Human Nutrition Research Center on Aging at Tufts University. They assessed both grip strength and gait speed and took measurements of blood concentrations of antioxidant levels (including vitamin C, vitamin E, and carotenoids). About 2,452 men and women, ages 33 to 88, underwent tests of walking speed and grip strength three times over several years. Higher intake of all antioxidants (except vitamin C) was associated with increased gait speed. Grip strength was better in those with higher amounts of total carotenoids, lycopene, and lutein plus zeaxanthin. Though the changes were modest, researchers state that small differences over time can be clinically meaningful and show that antioxidants highlight a protective effect against the loss of muscle and physical function in older adults.
American Journal of Clinical Nutrition, Nov. 12, 2020

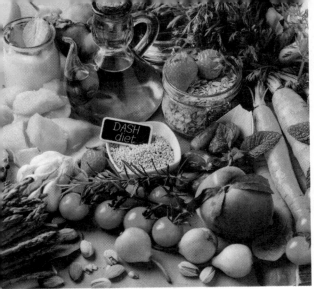
© Aamulya | Dreamstime

While the DASH diet was formulated to help with hypertension, its health benefits are far more reaching, and the diet's recommendations include a wide variety of foods, all focused on nutrition and health.

in olive oil have beneficial health effects, as do the high levels of antioxidant phytochemicals.

The potential anti-inflammatory effects of the Mediterranean-style dietary pattern are thought to be responsible for its health benefits. This way of eating has been associated with the prevention of cardiovascular disease, type 2 diabetes, atrial fibrillation, and breast cancer. Following a Mediterranean dietary pattern can lower cholesterol and triglyceride levels; protect against oxidative stress, inflammation, and blood clotting; modify hormones and growth factors involved in cancer; and support the health of gut microbiota that influence our metabolic health.

The Mediterranean diet also has been linked to a decreased risk of macular degeneration, dementia, and metabolic syndrome, which is a cluster of health problems that includes high blood pressure, elevated blood sugar, abnormal blood cholesterol and triglycerides, and excess abdominal fat. If you have three or more of these health problems, your risk for heart disease and type 2 diabetes is high.

The DASH Plan

Nearly half of American adults have high blood pressure (hypertension), according to the Centers for Disease Control and Prevention (CDC). If you're one of them, you may want to consider a hypertension diet in line with the Dietary Approaches to Stop Hypertension (DASH) pattern—a diet plan recognized to lower blood pressure. However, the DASH dietary pattern is not just for people with high blood pressure; it is an overall healthy choice for anyone.

As with other healthy dietary patterns, DASH recommendations include eating plenty of fruits, vegetables, and whole grains; adding nuts, seeds, and legumes several times a week; keeping dairy products low-fat or fat-free and meats lean; and limiting fats, oils, sweets, and added sugars. DASH emphasizes limiting sodium to under 2,300 milligrams (mg) per day, in addition to focusing on eating plenty of foods rich in nutrients that help to lower blood pressure, including potassium, magnesium, and calcium.

Research shows that the DASH diet may help lower stroke risk by reducing plaque buildup in the arteries. Additionally, DASH may slow the progression of both heart and kidney disease.

Plant-Based Diets

Research clearly associates a diet high in plant foods (like fruits, vegetables, whole grains, and beans) and low in meats with better health. The Meatless Monday campaign, in association with the Johns Hopkins' Bloomberg School of Public Health (meatlessmonday.com), reports that going meatless even one day a week will not only reduce cancer and heart-disease risk, fight diabetes, curb obesity, and increase lifespan, it also will support the environment by reducing carbon footprints and water usage and by decreasing our dependence on fossil fuels.

Whether you're a vegetarian (avoiding meat, but still eating eggs and dairy), a vegan (eschewing all animal products), or a pescatarian (including fish and seafood in an otherwise vegetarian or vegan diet), it's entirely possible to fuel your body for good health, with plenty of energy for exercise left over.

The good news is that you don't have to be perfect all the time to reap benefits from good nutrition, and a dietary pattern can (and should) be tailored to your personal tastes, preferences, schedule, budget, and current health needs. It needs to fit you to work.

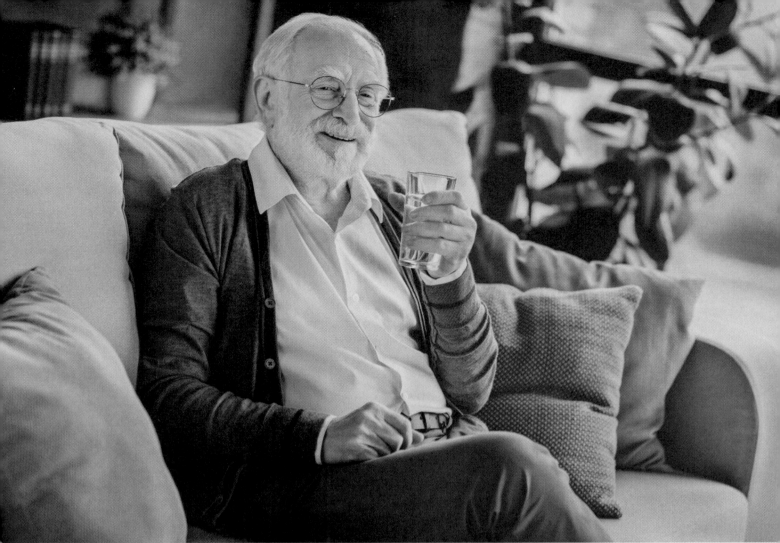

4 Hydration and Health

Why is hydration crucial to human health? About 60 percent of your body is composed of water. It is needed to deliver nutrients and oxygen to cells, to assist digestion, control blood pressure, and regulate body temperature. Not enough water can induce headaches and make a person dizzy, confused, and weak. It can also affect your attention, focus, reasoning, and motor coordination.

While many foods contain fluids and do provide the body some hydration, water is the ideal choice to stay hydrated. Recommended daily amounts vary, depending on health status, what you do, and where you live. Also, you age, the ability to sense thirst declines, so it's important to make drinking water a part of your daily health habit. A good way to start is to simply fill a pitcher with about 64 ounces of water and drink it throughout the day.

Of course, water choices vary. There's tap, filtered, and spring, just to name a few. Sales of bottled water have been rising for years. Bottlers sell billions of dollars of water annually. But as most consumers realize, bottled water, especially in plastic, comes at a cost financially and environmentally. Research suggests that chemicals from plastics could be leaching into the water that people drink. Of concern is bisphenol A, also known as BPA, which is pervasive in our environment (e.g., plastic wrap, cans lined with BPA epoxy resin, and

The need for adequate hydration is not just an athletic requirement. Your body needs about 96 ounces (for women) to 128 ounces (for men) of water per day. But, as you will learn in this chapter, 20 to 30 percent of it can come from food.

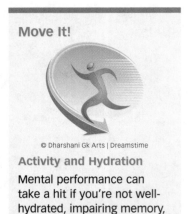

© Dharshani Gk Arts | Dreamstime

Activity and Hydration

Mental performance can take a hit if you're not well-hydrated, impairing memory, math skills, and mood.

Hydrating Fruits and Vegetables

Fruits and vegetables top the list of water-rich foods, whether raw or cooked. This sampling shows the percentage of water (by weight) in common fruits and vegetables.

FOOD	PERCENT WATER
cucumbers	96
zucchini, cooked	95
cherry tomatoes	94
romaine lettuce	94
sweet red peppers	92
spinach	91
strawberries	91
watermelon	91
peaches	89
carrots	88
oranges	86
pineapples	86
apples	85
pears	84
mangos	83
grapes	81
bananas	75

Source: USDA National Nutrient Database. Values for all fruits are fresh, raw unless marked cooked.

plastic containers). BPA may mimic or interfere with hormones such as estrogen, androgens, and thyroid hormones. Though there's little definitive data on the impact to humans, as of 2018, the U.S. Food & Drug administration banned the use of BPA in baby bottles and baby sipping cups.

In reality, a lot of packaged bottled water is just purified tap water that has been filtered in similar ways that you can do at home. Reverse osmosis filters that fit under the sink and filters that fit on faucets or in pitchers do a decent job of filtering trace contaminants. Reusable metal or glass containers can save you money and spare the environment from plastic trash. It's estimated that up to 86 percent of plastic water bottles end up in the trash or as litter.

Finally, be aware of unverified health claims about alkaline or electrolyte-enhanced waters. Alkaline waters do contain higher pH levels compared to most tap or bottled waters, and proponents claim they help keep the body in balance, but there's little evidence to back this up. Electrolyte waters contain added minerals, such as sodium, potassium, and magnesium. But unless you sweat profusely or are severely dehydrated, these products aren't really necessary for everyday hydration.

Read on to discover more about how much fluid you need, how to know if you are becoming dehydrated, and the best food and beverage choices to help you maintain hydration.

What Your Body Needs

The general rule of thumb is to drink at least eight 8-ounce glasses (for 64 ounces) of water per day. But your individual needs depend on a lot of factors, including the weather and your activities. Your body size and gender also figure in to how much fluid you need daily.

The Dietary Reference Intakes from the U.S. National Academy of Science's Institute of Medicine say that the Adequate Intake Level (which covers the needs of most people) for water is 12 cups (96 ounces) per day for women and 16 cups (128 ounces) per day for men, but you don't need to drink that much, because an estimated 20 to 30 percent of this amount comes from the foods you eat.

Fruits and vegetables contain varying amounts of water. For example, cucumber, watermelon, and zucchini are high in water. But other foods contribute to water intake, too. Soup, cooked cereal, and even some foods you might not think of as containing water, such as cooked brown rice or pasta, fish, poultry, and eggs, contain water to help you hydrate (see "Hydrating Fruits and Vegetables").

Consequences of Dehydration

A more common problem than hyponatremia is dehydration, which occurs when your fluid losses (through sweating and urination) exceed fluid intake. Dehydration can contribute to many common health concerns, such as constipation, falls, urinary-tract infections, and kidney stones.

Mental performance takes a hit when you're dehydrated, too: Dehydration can impair memory, math ability, and mood. It also can hinder the mental activity needed to support physical movement and hand-eye coordination. Emerging evidence suggests dehydration may increase the risk of free-radical damage in the body's cells and tissues, which can contribute to chronic-disease risk. Excessive dehydration during prolonged exercise can place greater demands on the cardiovascular system and increase a person's risk for heat-related illness (e.g., heat exhaustion, heat stroke).

People who don't get enough sleep also may risk the effects of dehydration. Researchers from Pennsylvania State University learned that a hormone called vasopressin, which helps regulate hydration status, was disrupted in study participants who had less than six hours of sleep. The 2018 study suggests that if you're not getting enough sleep and you feel tired the next day, drink extra water as you could be dehydrated.

Obviously, the risk of dehydration increases with intense physical activity since water leaving the body as sweat is produced to dissipate heat. Certain disease states, such as diabetes and hypertension (high blood pressure), also can increase risk. In some cases, dehydration is partly due to medications, such as diuretics and laxatives, used to treat health conditions.

The water for sweat comes partly from your blood, so when you become dehydrated, the volume of blood circulating through your body decreases, your blood becomes thicker, and blood flow can become compromised. As a result, your blood is less able to deliver oxygen to muscles, carry away waste materials, and help rid the body of excess heat.

At the same time, your heart rate increases to help push the blood to your muscles and vital organs, such as your brain and lungs. For every 1 percent of body weight lost due to dehydration, heart rate increases by five to eight beats per minute and core body temperature increases by 0.18° to 0.72°F.

Warning Signs. Symptoms that indicate dehydration include thirst, dizziness or lightheadedness, dry mouth, unusual fatigue, unusually rapid heartbeat, headache, and infrequent urination. You can purchase wearable products that can track your hydration status in real time, but you can still use lower-tech methods to keep tabs on your hydration:

Urine Color. The idea is that if your urine is pale yellow (looks like lemonade), you're well-hydrated. If your urine is darkly colored (looks like apple juice) and limited in volume, you may be inadequately hydrated.

Several factors can interfere with the results, however. For example, some medications and vitamin supplements can discolor urine. Certain foods, such as beets and rhubarb, can temporarily discolor urine in some people, too.

Weight Fluctuations. If you weigh yourself first thing every morning after urinating and your body weight fluctuates by less than 1 percent from day to day, it's a sign you're adequately hydrated. Similarly, if you weigh yourself before and after exercise, it can give you an idea of your hydration status, assuming you began exercise well-hydrated. A decrease in body weight between 3 and 5 percent after exercise represents significant dehydration.

Overhydration. Referred to as overhydration, drinking too much water can lead to hyponatremia. Symptoms of hyponatremia include headache, confusion, dizziness, nausea and/or vomiting, weight gain, muscle cramps, and weakness; in some cases, hyponatremia can be a serious life-threatening condition.

Choosing Fluids

Staying well-hydrated is important, but what you choose to drink to stay hydrated can have a big impact on other facets of your health.

As already emphasized, water generally is the best choice for quenching thirst and staying hydrated. Any fluid you drink contains water, but choosing plain water hydrates without calories, sugars,

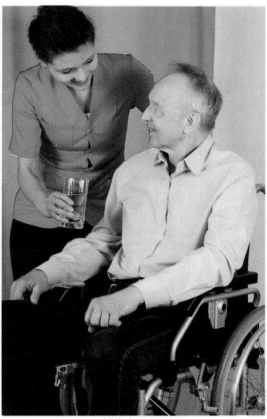

© Bialasiewicz | Dreamstime

Elderly adults often have an impaired thirst mechanism and therefore may lack the sensation of thirst. If you're a caregiver, be sure to periodically encourage people to drink some water.

food coloring, or additives. If plain water doesn't excite you, add some fun to that water (see "Make Water Exciting").

The next few sections look at some other healthful fluid choices (milk, coffee, and tea), some that should be avoided (sugary beverages and energy drinks), and others that fall somewhere in between (sports drinks and fruit juices). See "Alcohol Risks."

(see "Make Water Exciting").

See "Alcohol Risks."

Make Water Exciting

Add some fun to that water glass! Wash fruits and vegetables (including the peel), as well as fresh herbs, first. Add several pieces of your favorite flavoring agent(s) to a pitcher of water, bruise (squeeze) them a bit to release the flavor, and refrigerate for at least two hours, or ideally, overnight, to allow the flavors to infuse into the water. Try flavor combinations, such as watermelon-basil, blueberry-lemon, or cucumber-mint. Consider trying:

- basil leaves
- berries
- cucumber slices
- orange, lemon, lime, and grapefruit slices
- grapes
- herbal-tea bags
- kiwi slices
- mango slices
- mint leaves
- peach slices
- pineapple slices
- rosemary sprigs
- sage leaves
- sweet cherries, pitted
- watermelon cubes, seedless

Alcohol Risks

To reduce the risk of alcohol-related harms, the *2020–2025 Dietary Guidelines for Americans* recommends that adults of legal drinking age can choose not to drink, or to drink in moderation by limiting intake to two drinks or less in a day for men or one drink or less in a day for women, on days when alcohol is consumed. A "drink" is equivalent to 12 fluid ounces of a 5 percent alcohol beer, 5 fluid ounces of wine (12 percent alcohol), or 1.5 fluid ounces of 80 proof distilled spirits (40 percent alcohol).

Alcoholic beverages should be avoided right before exercise. Alcohol acts as a diuretic by inhibiting the production of a hormone that tells your body to hold onto water, thus contributing to dehydration. Alcohol also impairs judgment and balance and slows reflexes. It can suppress the use of body fat to fuel exercise, too.

Excess drinking of alcohol during the day prior to exercise may impair performance, even though blood alcohol concentration is zero when you start exercising. The effects of alcohol on strength and performance may continue for several hours after signs of intoxication or a hangover go away.

Although it may be tempting to celebrate with alcohol after an athletic competition, it could contribute to further water loss from the body. Beverages with high alcohol concentrations, such as hard liquor, have a significant diuretic effect and should not be used when you're trying to rehydrate quickly. Wine may be problematic as well.

The alcohol concentrations in a typical beer (4 to 4.5 percent) may not interfere with hydration over the long-term in active people, but they aren't a good choice when you're trying to rehydrate quickly (and beware of higher alcohol brews or "craft beers").

Besides interfering with rehydration, alcohol may interfere with post-exercise recovery by impairing storage of glucose and delaying muscle repair.

Regardless of when alcohol is consumed, it can decrease your vitamin and mineral absorption, thus increasing your risk of deficiency. Alcohol also adds unneeded empty calories, especially if consumed regularly.

Plant-Based and Dairy Milks

Milk supplies the body with fluid to stay hydrated, and it provides protein to satisfy appetite and support muscles and calcium to help maintain strong bones. Most commercial milk products are fortified with vitamin D to improve calcium absorption as well.

Dairy is a source of saturated fat, however, and has been associated with an increased risk for cardiovascular disease. That's why experts recommend using low-fat or non-fat (skim) milk for drinking and cooking for anyone over 2 years of age. A 2020 study also suggested that full-fat milk may negatively affect aging. Researchers from Brigham Young University reported telomeres were shorter in the adults studied who consumed higher-fat milk compared to those who drank lower-fat milk. Telomeres are the nucleotide endcaps of human chromosomes. They act like a biological clock and are correlated with age.

Many adults don't have enough of the enzyme lactase to properly digest the milk-sugar lactose. If you get a bellyache or digestive upset after eating or drinking dairy products, you may be lactose intolerant. Options for putting milk back in your diet—including enzyme pills that can be taken before ingesting dairy, enzyme drops that can be added to liquid dairy, and milks with the lactose already broken down, such as Lactaid—can help you.

You may also be interested in A2 milk. The designation "A2" refers to a form of beta-casein protein in the milk. According to the California Dairy Research Foundation, the typical dairy cow in the United States produces approximately equal amounts of A1 and A2 forms of beta-casein in its milk. Other types of cows are naturally more likely to produce only A2 proteins. While good-quality research in humans is limited at this time, it has been proposed that some people who think they are lactose-intolerant are reacting to A1 proteins and would be better able to tolerate milk containing only the A2 form of the protein.

For those who prefer to skip dairy altogether, there are a wide variety of plant "milks" on the market. Be aware that, except for soymilk, most of these milks have a lot less protein, so they do not take the place of cow's milk in the diet (if you're drinking cow's milk for protein reasons). Make sure that any product you choose is calcium-fortified, and check labels to avoid added sugars.

Coffee and Tea

Coffee and tea are two of the most popular beverages worldwide. Both have been the subject of many studies, some of which suggest that these beverages may provide a variety of health benefits.

Coffee is rich in many beneficial compounds, such as health-promoting phytochemicals, enzymatic reaction-activating magnesium, and antioxidant lignans. Such compounds may contribute to the benefits associated with coffee drinking, including lower risks of stroke, arterial plaque (atherosclerosis), type 2 diabetes, depression, Parkinson's disease, and Alzheimer's disease, as well as improved longevity. In addition, the health benefits of decaffeinated coffee are largely similar to those found in coffee with caffeine.

Watch out for the sugars and fat that are commonly added to coffee drinks, however. The negative effects of these tasty additions may outweigh the benefits of the coffee itself.

Tea is also full of health-promoting compounds. Black, green, white, and oolong tea all come from the leaves of the same plant, *Camellia sinensis*, which is rich in antioxidant flavonoids, but the

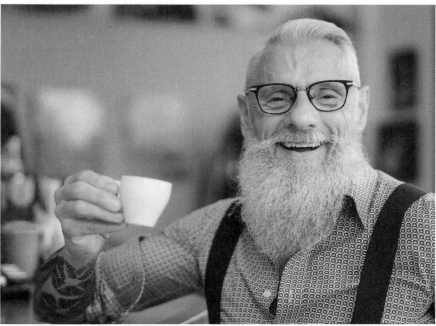

Coffee is rich in phytochemicals, which are good for you!

different teas vary in the ways the leaves are processed. Drinking a cup of tea may provide you with as large a dose of antioxidant flavonoids as a serving of flavonoid-rich fruits and vegetables.

Given tea's antioxidant content, it may come as no surprise that an analysis of several studies found that drinking three cups of tea daily was associated with an 11 percent drop in the risk of heart attacks. Other studies have linked green tea to better blood cholesterol and triglyceride levels. Interestingly, countries with the highest rates of black-tea consumption have lower rates of type 2 diabetes. Regular tea drinking also has been linked with a reduced risk of certain cancers and may support better brain function with age.

Herbal teas are not teas at all since they don't contain leaves from the tea plant. Instead, they are an infusion or blend of leaves, fruits, bark, roots, or flowers of other plants. These tasty brews are caffeine-free and have natural flavors that may be more appealing to people who find true teas bitter.

While packages of so-called functional teas boast health benefits like weight loss, reduction of anxiety, and boosting of

Nutrition Facts

8 servings per container
Serving size   2/3 cup (55g)

Amount per serving

Calories   230

	% Daily Value*
Total Fat 8g	10%
Saturated Fat 1g	5%
Trans Fat 0g	
Cholesterol 0mg	0%
Sodium 160mg	7%
Total Carbohydrate 37g	13%
Dietary Fiber 4g	14%
Total Sugars 12g	
Includes 10g Added Sugars	20%
Protein 3g	
Vitamin D 2mcg	10%
Calcium 260mg	20%
Iron 8mg	45%
Potassium 240mg	6%

* The % Daily Value (DV) tells you how much a nutrient in a serving of food contributes to a daily diet. 2,000 calories a day is used for general nutrition advice.

Read those food labels. It can be astonishing how much added sugar is found in commercial foods. Fruit can satisfy your sweet tooth and offers fiber and other important nutrients.

immune function, none of these statements have been evaluated by the FDA, and solid data on these health effects is limited. Some research shows that a few herbal teas, like chamomile and valerian, may have the potential to reduce anxiety and improve sleep.

A 2014 study published in *PLOS One* found that drinking caffeinated beverages does not interfere with hydration in people who habitually drink moderate amounts of caffeinated beverages.

Regularly consuming caffeine may lead to tolerance against its diuretic effect. If you're not used to drinking caffeinated beverages, they would not be a good choice before exercise, not only because of the possible diuretic effect, but also due to their potential to make you feel jittery.

Beware of Added Sugars

Sugar-sweetened beverages (SSBs) supply around half of the added sugars in the American diet. This non-diet drink category includes regular soda, lemonade, fruit punch, sports drinks, energy drinks, flavored milks, most iced teas, and coffee drinks. These beverages provide "empty calories" with little-to-no nutritional value.

The intake of added sugars is associated with a growing list of health problems, and SSBs themselves have been linked to weight gain, obesity, heart disease, type 2 diabetes, gout, fatty liver, and a host of metabolic risk factors (including increased triglycerides, high blood pressure, and insulin resistance). Sugary sodas may even cause you to age faster, causing inflammation and promoting DNA changes associated with aging.

Although you could replace sugar-sweetened beverages with artificially sweetened ones to save calories, some studies suggest that the intense sweetness of sugar substitutes may foster a greater preference for sweets and increase your appetite for them. They certainly do nothing to combat our preference for sweet foods. Research suggests people who drink diet soda are more likely to make less healthful food choices, which is counterproductive to achieving good health. If you choose to drink diet soda to satisfy your sweet tooth or transition away from regular sodas, do so in moderation.

Sports/Energy Drinks

If you're sweating lightly or exercising for an hour or less, plain water works just fine for hydrating, and special electrolyte-replacement drinks are not necessary. Despite this fact, sports drinks such as Gatorade and Powerade are frequently used. These drinks add sweeteners to replenish energy burned in exercise and enhance taste, electrolytes (primarily sodium and a bit of potassium) to replace those lost in sweat, and food coloring to make them visually appealing. Like other sugar-sweetened beverages, sports drinks can increase the risk of tooth enamel erosion and dental decay. They also may contribute to weight gain, and added sugars are known to increase heart-disease risk. Stick to water unless you are exercising long and hard.

If you are doing endurance or high-intensity aerobic exercise for more than one hour or lower-intensity exercise for longer periods, carbohydrate consumption (such as from most sports drinks) can help sustain and improve your exercise performance. If you are exercising at this level, try one-half to one liter of a sports drink each hour to maintain hydration.

Sports drinks should not be confused with energy drinks, such as Red Bull, Monster, and Rockstar. Energy drinks contain caffeine and sometimes other purported energy boosters, such as guarana (which has twice the caffeine of coffee beans) and taurine (which boosts caffeine's effects), not to mention sugar—more than 13 teaspoons (52 grams) in a 16-ounce can. These drinks are not designed to be fluid-replacement beverages, and there is little scientific evidence to support the idea that they improve sports performance.

There are plenty of reasons to avoid energy drinks. Preliminary evidence shows energy drinks raise blood pressure in healthy adults compared with similar drinks formulated without caffeine and other stimulants. The acidic drinks also can harm teeth, and the stimulants may contribute to anxiety and sleep problems.

Most worrisome is research showing that there are a substantially increasing number of emergency-room visits each year involving energy drinks, and the number of these visits involving adults over 40 grew dramatically during the study period. It is possible that energy-drink components may interact with prescription medications.

Sugary Fruit Drinks

Beware of sugar water masquerading as fruit juice. To earn the title "fruit juice," a product must contain undiluted fruit juice (although it can have added sugar). A fruit beverage, drink, cocktail, or punch typically contains little fruit juice.

Fruit juice that is labeled "100% juice" has some of the vitamins, minerals, and phytochemicals from the whole fruit, along with the sugars, but not the fiber to slow down the release of those sugars into the bloodstream. Limit even 100 percent fruit juice to around 8 ounces a day and consider diluting it with water.

Hydration Plan for Exercise

When you're preoccupied with physical activity, you may not think about the fact that you're thirsty. Even if you do tap into your thirst level, fluid may not be readily available unless you plan ahead. So, it's important to hydrate before exercise,

plan for hydration during longer and/or more vigorous exercise sessions, and rehydrate afterward.

For guidance on hydration, see "Exercise Hydration Guidelines." When you go into exercise adequately hydrated, you are more likely to have a lower core body temperature and heart rate during exercise.

The environment in which you're exercising can have a big impact on fluid in your body. For example, heat, humidity, and high altitudes all cause fluid loss and increase your body's need for water. In hot weather, a 10°F increase in temperature can cause a 50 to 60 percent increase in water requirements at rest. If you're exercising or working hard in such hot-weather conditions, your water needs will increase well beyond this amount.

High relative humidity (the water content of the air) is also a problem. Sweat evaporating off the skin lowers body temperature. If the air is already saturated with water (high humidity), the sweat won't evaporate as effectively, and this natural thermoregulation system can't work.

Although you may not think about water loss when you're exercising at a high altitude in colder weather, you lose about twice the amount of water just through breathing than you would at sea level. Because there's less oxygen in the air at higher altitudes, you naturally breathe deeper and more rapidly.

Additionally, when you're exercising in cold conditions, your sense of thirst is blunted, and you may not think to hydrate as often as you would in hot-weather conditions. Remember, you may sweat more if you over-dress in cold weather, and cold weather may trigger increased urination, so be especially aware of hydration in such conditions, especially if you're not acclimated to them.

Exercise Hydration Guidelines

Follow these guidelines to avoid under- or over-hydration when exercising:

Before Exercise

- Drink 16 to 20 fluid ounces (2 to 2½ cups) at least four hours before exercise.
- Drink 2 to 8 fluid ounces (¼ to 1 cup) of water 10 to 15 minutes before exercise.

During Exercise

- When exercising less than 60 minutes, water is all that is needed.
- When exercising more than 60 minutes, drink 3 to 8 fluid ounces of water or a sports beverage (5 to 8 percent carbohydrate with electrolytes) every 15 to 20 minutes.
- Do not drink more than 1 quart (32 ounces) per hour.
- For lengthy activity, such as hiking or a long bike ride outdoors, wear a bottle belt, and always carry money with you in case you need to buy a beverage.

After Exercise

- Weigh yourself right before and after activity (prior to drinking or urinating). If you've lost less than one pound during exercise, you've done a good job of staying hydrated.
- Drink 20 to 24 fluid ounces of water or a sports beverage for every pound of weight lost during exercise. The goal is to correct your losses within two hours after exercise.
- Do not consume more than 1 liter (33.8 ounces) of fluid per hour. Overhydration, also called water intoxication, can result in behavioral changes, confusion, drowsiness, nausea/vomiting, muscle cramps, weakness/paralysis, and a risk of death.

Source: American College of Sports Medicine Information on Selecting and Effectively Using Hydration for Fitness.

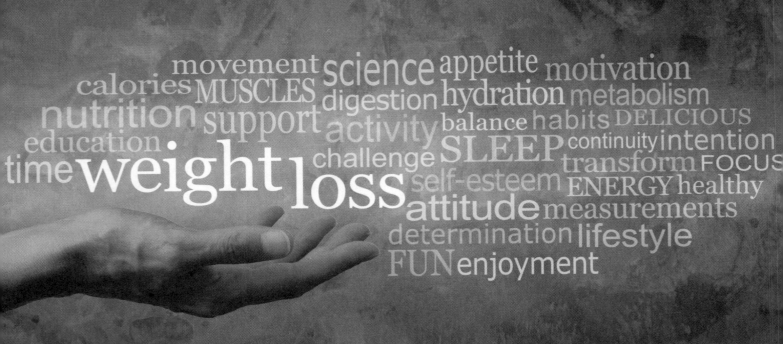

Healthy food and regular exercise naturally help maintain normal body weight.

5 Weight Loss Without Struggle

Weight loss is something a lot of people struggle with, often for their entire lives. Sure a few pounds might be lost here and there, but it's frequently regained. That's because the habit of healthy eating per an individual's specific needs may have never been fully formed. But if you break down obstacles to success and look to the power of habits, there is a new opportunity.

Eating while doing something else is a habit for many people. It may have started in childhood when many people's eyes were glued to a cereal box. Now, you may wolf down a large bag of buttery low-calorie popcorn while binge-watching videos or finish an entire pint of gelato while scrolling through social media.

Habits can better serve our health or spoil it. For example, brushing your teeth every morning and night is good. A midnight snack of leftover fast-food, not so much. But learn to harness the unconscious nature of habits for good and you can accelerate success in virtually any domain you desire, be it weight loss, weight maintenance, improved nutrition, or more physical activity.

The Secret Power of Habits

When habits are fully formed, we barely think about them. And that's their inherent beauty and power. They become mindless because there's no willpower involved. For example, you don't have to think about taking the toothpaste cap off, filling your toothbrush with paste, and moving the brush inside your mouth. It's basically automatic. It just happens. And when you hijack a habit to build another one, you're not wasting precious and limited willpower on trying to accomplish a task (see "How to Lose Weight").

How to Hack a Habit

Here's how hijacking habits can work. Many people have coffee first thing in the morning. Making the brew is automatic: same coffee, same amount, same process, every day. Add to that habit another goal. For example, maybe you want to drink more water. While the coffee is brewing or dripping, you set out your usual coffee cup. Add to that a large glass of water and drink it before you enjoy your coffee. Do that for several days, and soon downing an extra-large glass of water becomes routine. Similarly, if you find yourself starving in the late afternoon and default for an easy donut fix, use your morning coffee-making time to prep a healthy snack for later in the day. Eventually, drinking more water and eating a healthy afternoon snack become a habit. Both are expedited when desired goals are stacked onto existing habits.

On the flip side, breaking a bad habit can be more easily achieved when there's more friction to completing it. For example, to thwart nighttime TV munchies, don't buy the bag of buttery popcorn or gelato. When you turn on the TV, perhaps pick up a knitting needle, coloring book, or do your nails instead. Make it more difficult to consume the unwanted food (see "Healthy Habits Maintain Weight Loss").

How can you get started? First, take an assessment of your habits, both good and bad. Then get creative. Think of ways to hijack existing habits to create new ones, and place obstacles in front of those you'd like to break. And give it time. From repetition often comes affinity. We do come to like that which we may have not appreciated before. With some patience and persistence, new habits become an effortless reality and the spell of old ones can forever be broken. Slow and steady wins the race.

Smart Choices

Weight loss is not rocket science, but it does require smart choices and dedication to a healthy lifestyle for life. Sure, you can have occasional indulgences, but the keyword is "occasional." Following healthful dietary patterns like the ones outlined in Chapter 3 will make it more likely that weight loss is accompanied by good health.

There are no magic weight-loss foods, but there are ways of eating that will make weight loss easier, while ensuring you stay well-nourished and satisfied.

Portion Distortion

Research shows that people eat more when they are given larger portions. Unfortunately, portion sizes in the United States have grown tremendously.

How to Lose Weight

- **Eating habits must change.** A whopping 98 percent of participants in the National Weight Control Registry modified their food intake to lose weight.

- **Physical activity is key.** A full 94 percent increased their physical activity; 90 percent exercise an average of an hour a day. Walking was the most frequently reported form of activity, so gym memberships and personal trainers are not required.

- **Less screen time increases active time.** Most participants (62 percent) watch less than 10 hours of TV per week.

- **Weight-loss programs are not essential.** While 55 percent of registry participants used some type of weight-loss program, 45 percent lost the weight on their own.

- **Regular meals are important.** More than three-quarters of registry particpants report eating breakfast every day.

- **Tracking efforts helps.** While the scale is not for everyone, 75 percent of registry participants report weighing themselves at least once a week.

Source: The National Weight Control Registry

NEW FINDING

Healthy Habits Maintain Weight Loss

Researchers identified specific behavioral and psychological strategies that may help people who have lost weight keep it off. The study surveyed over 4,700 participants in a weight-loss program who had maintained a weight loss of at least 20 pounds for more than three years. A group of over 500 weight-stable individuals with obesity served as a control group. The weight-loss group reported more frequent, habitual, healthy dietary choices; greater self-monitoring; and the employment of psychological coping strategies. They were also more willing to ignore food cravings. Key strategies included keeping low-calorie foods accessible, setting daily calorie goals, daily recording of caloric intake, and regularly measuring foods. Specific psychological coping strategies included "thinking about past successes" and "remaining positive in the face of weight regain." Importantly, people for whom healthy eating became a habit had more success maintaining weight loss. While this study focused on individuals in one specific weight-loss program, these results are in line with other studies that indicate successful weight-loss maintainers generally eat a lower-calorie diet and have higher levels of physical activity, dietary restraint, and self-monitoring behaviors. Sustaining weight loss has been shown to maintain improvements in cardiometabolic risk factors.

Obesity, January 2020

According to the National Institutes of Health, portions have indeed become supersized in just a few decades. For example, about 20 years ago, a bagel was 3 inches in diameter and about 150 calories, but today bagels are typically 6 inches in diameter and 350 calories. At fast-food restaurants, containers of fries are about three times larger, sodas six times larger and burgers four times the size they used to be. Portions have indeed grown, and so have our waistlines. According to a 2020 Tufts University study, the typical American adult gets one of every five calories from a restaurant meal, and not only are portions excessively large, nutritional quality is sorely lacking. That doesn't mean you should never eat out, you just need to be smarter about it (see "Eating Out without Overeating").

And it's not just restaurant food that's adding to our waistlines. Bags are bigger, bowls are deeper, even the plates we eat from have increased in diameter! The plate depicted in MyPlate images is nine inches across; chances are the salad plates in your dish set are closer to that

Eating Out without Overeating

If you're like many Americans, you eat out at least three times a week and consume about a third of your calories away from home. Large portions and flavorful, calorie-dense dishes typically served at restaurants can hijack self-control and lead to excess intake, despite your best intentions. Although some people might think they'll compensate by eating less at other times, several studies show this generally doesn't occur. Additionally, as we grow accustomed to oversized portions served in restaurants, we may inadvertently increase portion sizes at home. Eating out three times a week adds up to more than 150 meals a year, so your choices could have a big impact on your health.

Fast Food: Look at the Calories

Eating fast food is linked with obesity, but other restaurant meals can be just as problematic when it comes to consuming excess calories, and food at non-chain restaurants is as caloric as food at chains. Susan Roberts, PhD, director of the Energy Metabolism Laboratory at Tufts University's Human Nutrition Research Center on Aging (HNRCA), and her colleagues analyzed the calorie content of 364 common dinners from the nine most popular cuisines in randomly selected non-chain restaurants in three large U.S. cities. They compared them with equivalent dishes from top-selling, large-chain restaurants. The non-chain meals averaged 1,205 calories, which was not significantly different from equivalent meals from large chains. American, Italian, and Chinese entrées were especially high in calories, averaging 1,495 calories per meal. To put that into perspective, an average adult may need 570 calories per meal or less, depending on age, activity level, body size, sex, eating frequency, and other factors. In this study, 92 percent of the meals analyzed had more than 570 calories.

Many restaurants are now required by law to list calories on their menus, but non-chain restaurants and small chains with less than 20 locations are not. Non-chain and small-chain eateries account for about 50 percent of restaurants in the United States.

Portion-Controlling at the Restaurant

It's not impossible to control your calories and make nutritious choices when eating out, but it does take effort and smart strategies. Follow these tips:

- **Research nutrition.** If you're considering going to a chain restaurant, check the restaurant's website for nutrition information. If it's a local, non-chain restaurant without nutrition information, check similar menu items on websites, such as calorieking.com, or in printed books of restaurant nutrition information. For help with meal options recommended by nutrition experts, try healthydiningfinder.com.

- **Find a healthier alternative.** If you're going out with a group, try to steer the choice to an eatery with smart choices, such as one that prepares a lot of fresh-fish dishes or leafy-green salads.

- **Rethink entrées and appetizers.** Multi-course meals are typically much more food than you need. Skip the appetizers or consider choosing an appetizer as a main course (since they're often a more reasonable size for a meal). Make ordering dessert a special treat and share it with the table. Choosing water or unsweetened tea also cuts calories and dramatically reduces the intake of added sugars.

- **Ask for substitutes.** If a sandwich comes with French fries, ask if you can substitute a simple vegetable that you see elsewhere on the menu. For breakfast, many places are happy to replace home fries with fruit, if you ask, although there may be an extra charge.

- **Request dressing on the side.** Dressings and dipping sauces typically add 100 to 200 calories to a dish, so ask for them on the side so you can control how much is used.

- **Half to go.** Once you dig into a dish, it can be difficult to stop nibbling, so minimize the temptation to overeat by taking half off your plate when it's served.

- **Share with a friend.** Splitting a meal with your companion is a great way to ensure you both eat a reasonable portion.

size than the dinner plates. Our brain is easily fooled: Eating food that fills a smaller plate is more satisfying than the same amount of food on a larger plate.

These tips will help you avoid some common portion-size pitfalls:

- **Use a plate:** Serve food on individual plates instead of putting the serving dishes on the table. Keeping the excess food out of reach may discourage overeating.
- **Mindful snacking:** When eating or snacking in front of the TV, put the amount that you plan to eat into a bowl or container. It's easy to overeat when your attention is focused on something else.
- **Avoid starvation:** If you feel hungry between meals, eat a healthy snack, like a piece of fruit or small salad, to avoid overeating at your next meal.
- **Divide and conquer:** The larger the package, the more people eat. Divide the contents of one large package into several smaller containers to help avoid over-consumption. Don't eat straight from the package. Instead, serve the food in a small bowl or container.
- **Out of sight and out of mind:** People tend to consume more when they have easy access to food. Put healthier foods front-and-center, and they'll get chosen more often. Keep a fruit bowl on the counter. If you must keep tempting foods like cookies, chips, or ice cream in the house, move them to a high shelf or the back of the freezer. Move the healthier foods to the front at eye level. When buying in bulk, store the excess in a place that's not too easy to get to, such as a high cabinet or at the back of the pantry.

Foods That Satisfy

Over the years, carbohydrate, protein, and fat have all been suggested as the food component in control of making us feel satisfied and stay satisfied. While there is research to support each one, protein has risen to the top as the most satisfying nutrient, followed by carbohydrate, and then fat (see "Forget the Fad Diets").

But these macronutrients are not alone in controlling our hungry/full signals. Micronutrients like calcium also play a role in control of our appetite. This may be because the body is designed to make sure it gets what it needs. When you're running low on an important nutrient like calcium, your body sends out a general signal that you're hungry.

Even non-nutrient food components get in on the act. Fiber, for example, will help you feel full longer. So, choosing naturally high-fiber foods like whole grains, vegetables, and fruits with your protein may allow you to eat more satisfying

Forget the Fad Diets

Diets that recommend severely restricting or eliminating entire food or nutrient groups (like low-carb diets) help with weight loss in the short term, but they can be difficult to follow long term, so weight-loss results generally don't last.

Without the recommended balance of carbohydrate, protein, and fat, it is difficult if not impossible to get all the nutrients you need. Cutting carbohydrates, for example, removes whole grains, calcium-rich dairy, fruits, and a wide variety of vegetables from your plate. Dietary patterns rich in these foods have been shown repeatedly to be associated with better health.

The best diet for health or weight loss is one that emphasizes plant foods and lean proteins in proportions that meet (but don't exceed) your healthy body weight calorie needs. Putting these health-promoting choices on your plate automatically edges out foods high in health-damaging refined grains, saturated fats, added sugars, and sodium.

There are many ways to construct a dietary pattern that suits your tastes and can help you meet your health goals, so make sure you choose a healthful option you can follow long-term. Use the proven dietary patterns discussed in this chapter as a guide and beware of trendy advice. One exception may be the intermittent fasting that is showing promise for numerous health benefits. Studies have shown that alternating between times of fasting and eating (intermittent fasting) supports cellular health, probably by triggering an age-old adaptation to periods of food scarcity called metabolic switching. Such a switch occurs when cells use up their stores of rapidly accessible, sugar-based fuel, and begin converting fat into energy in a slower metabolic process.

A 2019 study from the *New England Journal of Medicine* found that this way of eating improves blood sugar regulation, increases resistance to stress, suppresses inflammation, and decreases blood pressure, blood lipid levels, and resting heart rates. The approach focuses more on when to eat rather than strictly limiting what to eat. Intermittent fasting diets generally fall into two categories: daily time-restricted feeding, which narrows eating times to six to eight hours per day, and 5:2 intermittent fasting, in which people limit themselves to one moderate-sized meal two days each week.

meals, while still cutting calories.

One key to staying satisfied and well-nourished while watching caloric intake is to consider the energy density of your food. Energy density is the calories per gram of food. Foods with high energy density provide more calories per bite than foods with low energy density. Choosing low energy density foods allows you to take in fewer calories while eating the same amount of food in a day (see "Defining Energy Density").

A great way to make meals more filling and satisfying without adding extra calories is to add vegetables. Toss an extra helping of your favorites into stir fries, stews, chili, pasta dishes, and salads.

Pulses (beans, peas, and lentils), which provide both protein and fiber without a lot of calories, are a great addition to any meal. Pulses work well in chili, soup, or salad, or stirred into rice or pasta dishes to make them more nutritious and filling.

Outsmart Cravings

Choosing reasonable-sized portions of satisfying, healthful food will help you cut calories in a safe and healthy way. We are born knowing when we are hungry and when we are full, but years of ignoring those signals can cause us to lose the ability to recognize them. Multiple studies have linked eating quickly to being overweight, perhaps because slower eating tends to result in eating less (see "Take Charge and Create Success").

Mindful eating allows you to focus on what you are seeing, smelling, tasting, and feeling while you eat. This can improve food choices, support portion control, and increase enjoyment of food. Focus on what you are seeing, smelling, tasting, and feeling:

- **Pause before eating:** Ask yourself, "Do I really want this?" "What do I actually need in this moment?"
- **Sit down:** Don't eat at your desk. Try to eat at an uncluttered surface to reduce stress and decrease distractions. Don't work, read, watch TV, or use electronic devices while eating.
- **Take pleasure in your meal:** Be grateful for your food. Notice the color, texture, aroma, and flavor. Slow down and savor your meal.
- **Try new things:** Unfamiliar textures and flavors rekindle our interest in food and automatically cause us to slow down and taste our meal. (They also expand the range of our nutrient intake!)
- **Listen to yourself chewing:** A study found that we eat less when we can hear the food crunching.
- **Take a break:** Pause mid-meal and check in with yourself. Are you still truly hungry?

Defining Energy Density

Energy density refers to the number of calories in a specific amount of food. Foods with high energy density have more calories per bite than foods with low energy density. Since the fiber and fluid in foods like whole grains, fruits, and vegetables help make their energy density low, you can eat a larger, more satisfying meal with these nutritious choices than if you choose to get those same calories from nutrient-poor foods.

Both menus below are 1,800 calories	
MENU 1: UNHEALTHY More Energy Dense/ Nutrient Poor	**MENU 2: HEALTHY** Less Energy Dense/Nutrient Rich
This menu does not provide the recommended daily value (based on a 2000-calorie diet) of any major vitamin or mineral.	This menu provides over 100 percent of the daily value (based on a 2000-calorie diet) of most major vitamins and minerals.
BREAKFAST	**BREAKFAST**
• chocolate donut • 1 cup coffee • 1 tablespoon cream	• 2 hard-boiled eggs; 6 ounces nonfat plain Greek yogurt topped with ½ cup blueberries, 2 tablespoons walnuts, 2 tablespoons toasted wheat germ • 1 cup herbal tea
LUNCH	**LUNCH**
• cheeseburger • small order of French fries • 12 ounces cola	• leafy green main-dish salad with 4 cups spinach, 1 cup chopped tomato, ½ cup grated carrot, ½ cup green peas (frozen, thawed), ⅓ cup cubed avocado, ⅔ cup roasted diced chicken breast, 2 tablespoons pumpkin seeds, 1½ tablespoons vinegar-and-oil dressing • ⅔ cup low-fat (1 percent) cottage cheese • 3 rye crackers
DINNER	**DINNER**
• 2 slices pepperoni pizza • 1 ice cream sandwich	• 4 ounces broiled salmon, brushed with olive oil and drizzled with lemon juice • 1 cup quinoa • 7 spears broiled asparagus, brushed with oil • 3 fresh tomato slices with lemon juice • 1 cup sliced kiwifruit • 1 cup low-fat (1 percent) cow's milk

- **Adjust your environment:** If you can't banish the office candy jar, move it farther from your desk. Leave serving dishes off the table so you must get up for seconds. Alter your drive to work so you don't pass the donut shop at which you habitually stop.
- **Follow the "Rule of 2" when eating out:** Choose a reasonable entrée plus two other choices (salad and a vegetable, or bread and soup).
- **Save the best for last:** If the mashed potatoes are your favorite part of your meal, eat them last.
- **Make dessert a treat:** It's not an every-meal occurrence.
- **Don't deny; trust yourself:** A healthy dietary pattern doesn't mean never eating your favorites again. It means practicing moderation (how often and how much of these treats we indulge in) and slowing down to enjoy them.

The Hype of Superfoods

Some nutrient-rich foods are being called "superfoods" and are believed to be especially good for your health. Advertisers seem to be pushing new superfoods every day—from avocado to acai berries, and chia seeds to dark chocolate.

Each of these foods is high in at least one component that has been associated with good health, but none of them is the secret to a healthy life. Rather than focus on eating a lot of one food, it's better to take superfoods as representatives of health-promoting food categories.

For example, oats are a whole grain packed with fiber and nutrients, but other whole grains are nutrition powerhouses as well. Kale is a leafy green packed with vitamins, minerals, and health-promoting phytochemicals, but so are collard greens, chard, and spinach, to name just a few. Salmon is a great source of heart-healthy omega-3 fatty acids, but eating any fatty fish two times a week is associated with a lower risk for cardiovascular disease.

Take Charge and Create Success

It's easier to make good food choices when you don't have bad ones within reach. Stock your pantry and fridge with healthy choices; keep a bowl of fruit on the counter; change your route to work so you don't pass the donut shop; get rid of the candy bowl at work; propose monthly or quarterly office birthday parties to limit cake-filled days; lobby for healthy vending-machine choices; and replace large plates and bowls with smaller options. Don't feel you have to stock unhealthy snacks and desserts for children. Developing good habits at a young age is easier than breaking bad habits as an adult.

Remember that some things that seem unrelated to food may be getting in the way of your weight-loss efforts. Feeling tired could cause a craving for fast energy—in the unhealthy form of sugar and refined grains—so getting enough sleep is important when you're trying to control your appetite. Stay well-hydrated to prevent mistaking thirst for hunger. Be sure you don't skip meals or eat too late at night to help control blood sugar peaks and valleys, potentially reducing cravings and the desire to binge. As you will see in the next section, choosing to be physically active also plays an important role in healthy long-term weight loss.

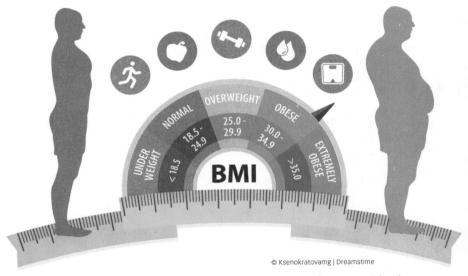

© Ksenokratovamg | Dreamstime

The consistent combination of a healthy diet and exercise can help you drop your body mass index, or BMI, the score health-care professionals use to measure healthy weight.

Avocados are packed with healthy fats as well, but those fats come with a high calorie count.

A lot of research has been done on blueberries, linking them to such benefits as a lower risk of dementia, but other berries provide the same family of phytochemicals and should have the same health benefits.

Enjoy the occasional piece of dark chocolate, but not simply for its antioxidants. Following a dietary pattern rich in a variety of fruits, vegetables, whole grains, and lean proteins like fish is the truly super way to reduce disease risk.

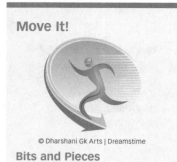
The Magic Combination

Exercising while you're cutting calories has benefits beyond burning calories. It's good for your heart, reduces stress, and helps muscles and bones stay strong. But many people believe that cutting calories alone will do the trick. Maybe. But you are better off adding that exercise component. Researchers in Taiwan attempted to determine the effects of dietary or exercise interventions, alone or combined, on weight loss in overweight or obese women. Not surprisingly, the authors found that dietary interventions reduce body weight and improve body composition in women more than exercise alone, but adding exercise reinforces the effect of the dietary interventions. And it makes you feel good, powerful, and strong. In addition, a lot of evidence supports the fact that exercise will prevent weight regain after successful weight loss.

Torch Calories

Aerobic exercise burns calories. The first step in building your exercise regimen is to aim for at least 150 minutes of moderate-intensity aerobic activity each week. To reach your weight goal, you may need to increase your activity beyond that. When it comes to maintaining weight loss and preventing weight regain over the long term, physical activity is needed.

Aerobic exercise can help you decrease body fat, including harmful abdominal fat. In fact, a weight-loss program that includes regular exercise preferentially reduces fat stored in the abdominal area, so if you've packed on excess fat around your middle, aerobic physical activity can help.

Many people overestimate how many calories they've burned during exercise and/or mistakenly think they need to refuel just because they've exercised. Both can interfere with your weight-control efforts.

Strengthen Muscles and Bones

When you lose weight, you can lose muscle and bone along with fat, but resistance (strength) training can help. Research studies have shown that:

- Any kind of regular exercise while cutting calories helps you lose more fat, but resistance training is better than aerobic exercise in helping you hold on to muscle.
- Performing resistance training while you cut calories may help prevent bone loss better than aerobic training.
- While resistance training alone will not lead to weight loss or improvement in health metrics like abdominal obesity, cholesterol, triglycerides, or blood pressure, resistance training plus cutting calories will.

Be aware that muscle weighs more than fat, so if you're gaining muscle while losing weight, the scale might not change as much as you'd like it to. The fit of your clothes is a better way to judge weight loss than the number on the scale.

Embrace Activity

If you're obese without other limiting disease conditions and your doctor has cleared you for exercise, standard exercise routines may be appropriate, although if it's been a long time since you've exercised, you will need to ease into it.

The *Physical Activity Guidelines for Americans* advise that obese individuals should work toward accumulating at least 150 to 300 minutes per week of moderate-intensity aerobic activity to help meet their weight goals. In some cases, two or more shorter sessions a day may be better tolerated and can help you reach this goal more easily.

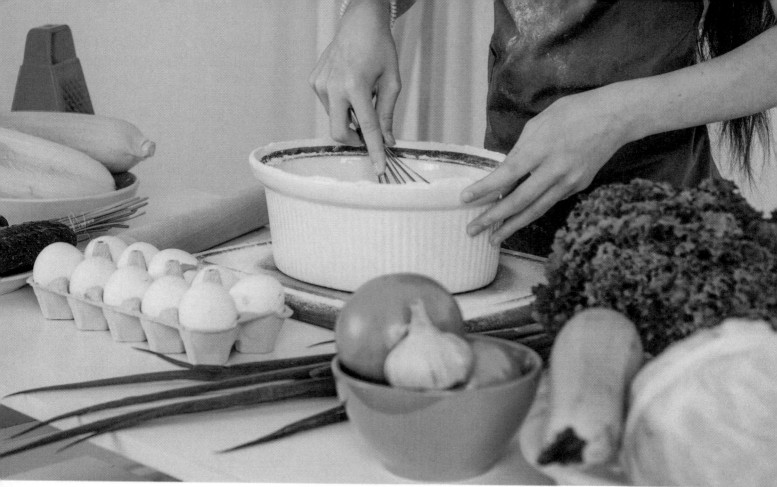

© Photosvit | Dreamstime

Having all your ingredients out, ready, and organized will make preparing a healthy meal much simpler.

6 Cooking Like a Pro

The French culinary term *mise en place* means "everything in its place." If you've watched a cooking show, you've seen this setup—small bowls and ramekins filled with all the ingredients neatly measured out and arranged in order of use. Apply this same concept in your kitchen and trying new recipes will become easier (and more successful). Having everything ready to go will also make cooking more efficient.

Preparation is the biggest difference between cooking like a pro or an amateur. A pro prepares and pays attention to details. In addition to the obvious ingredients, have all the needed items ready to go (e.g., knives, cutting boards, containers). Some dishes may require paper towels for drying ingredients and cleaners for decontaminating work surfaces along the way. Some people designate cutting boards for specific ingredients, one for veggies, another for meats, and perhaps a separate board for onions, garlic, and other alliums.

Consider the order in which you will prep ingredients. For example, if you need to clean mushrooms, arrange containers around the cutting board from left to right, one that holds the cleaned mushrooms, the middle container to catch the waste, and the third to hold the finished mushrooms. Break each job down into simple steps and think about efficiency of movement. When peeling carrots, for example, don't peel and cut each one. It's faster to peel them all and then cut them all.

Learn from the Pros

Taking a cooking class to learn pro tips can be a worthwhile investment and a fun activity, too. Some people get quite excited about taking a knife skills class. Learning how to safely chop, slice, and dice and which knives are best for a particular job is useful to everything you may do. There are many options online, but if it's possible to attend a live class, the instructor can provide more specific tips and answer individual questions. It's best to take a participatory class rather than just watching someone.

Consider creating a party around a theme (e.g., basic cooking skills, knife skills, or target a particular dish or cuisine). Hire a pro for a house party and invite people to join you. Involving other people in the process is an excellent opportunity to socialize and learn together. Involving people you live with or frequently see can extend the experience into cooking together on other days.

When everyone is invested in preparing a meal, there may be less resistance to trying something new, and there's value in understanding what it takes to prepare healthy, nutritious dishes. Yes, it takes time, but learning basic cooking skills from pros also can help you save time and money. Not every dish requires tons of ingredients and prep. In fact, with the right know how, you'll discover how to transform a few ingredients into a gourmet experience.

Creativity in the Kitchen

Eating well can be an exciting adventure. The world is your oyster! From African to Asian, barbecue to vegan, it all starts with the decision to try and is actualized by creating a plan. Host healthy potluck dinners, swap recipes with friends, or create your own healthy-chef challenge featuring an interesting basket of veggies.

It's easy to travel the world by stocking your kitchen with the right staples. Consider a humble plate of potatoes, zucchini, and carrots. Dress it with olive oil (fat), sea salt (salt), balsamic vinegar (acid), and lightly sauté (heat) those veggies. On another night, swap the olive oil for sesame oil, use miso (fermented soybean paste) as the salt, and quickly stir-fry.

Start with Whole Foods

Nutrition experts agree that eating whole foods is the best way to get the nutrients you need. Swap a cookie for diced pineapple or peaches drizzled with low-fat Greek yogurt, ditch the crackers and eat baked spicy sweet potatoes or herbed grilled veggies instead. These choices alone may help reduce the risk of heart disease. Switching from butter to vegetable oils, which are higher in heart-healthy unsaturated fats, is a smart choice. Try eating meatless meals once or twice a week (see "Plant-Based Eating"). All these ideas are relatively small changes with potentially big health impacts.

Here are a few more inspiring ways to transition to a healthier dietary pattern:

▸ **Whole-grain goodness.** Replace pasta, potatoes, and white rice with brown rice, barley, bulgur, quinoa, wheat berries, Kamut, and other tasty whole grains. All grains are cooked the same

---

Plant-Based Eating

A dietary pattern that emphasizes more plant foods and fewer animal foods may help reduce the risk of many common health problems, such as obesity, high blood pressure, heart disease, cancer, and diabetes, and it may help you live longer.

Cutting out animal products, however, removes a major source of protein in the Western diet. Fortunately, plant foods like beans, lentils, nuts, and even some grains can provide the protein you need. Although French fries, donuts, and soft drinks align with a plant-based diet, they're far from healthy.

Adding a salad to your daily routine and snacking on nuts and hummus are steps in the right direction, but many non-Western diets offer an amazing array of fabulous flavors just waiting to be explored. Chinese vegetable stir-fries and tofu dishes may be familiar to many, but the fresh tastes of Vietnamese cooking, the lentil dal in Indian food, bean dishes in Mexican cooking, and the chickpea-based hummus and falafel from the Mediterranean region are just a few examples of plant-based options to explore. Try some ideas from a vegetarian or vegan cookbook that appeal to you or use the many free websites or the vegetarian sections of popular recipe resources on the internet.

Adding more plant foods is a healthy choice, but you may want to consider working some animal-free meals into your repertoire. Use the Meatless Monday website for ideas on how to cut back on meat (see "A Better Burger?").

way: Put them in a pan with water or broth, bring to a boil, then simmer until the grain becomes tender. Grains can be cooked ahead and stored in the refrigerator for convenience. Check The Whole Grains Council website for more ideas (wholegrainscouncil.org).

- **Sugar-free and sweet.** Choose breakfast cereals with less than 10 grams of sugar and try cooking oatmeal with grated apple or chopped dates or top it with sliced bananas to sweeten without adding sugar. Replace sodas with water or unsweetened teas or make a refreshing spritzer by adding a splash of 100 percent fruit juice to the seltzer.
- **Fruit for dessert.** Make fruit your go-to dessert for when you crave something sweet. Fruit is as packed with nutrients as vegetables, and its sweetness helps scratch that sugar itch without nutrition-empty calories. Bake apples or try topping grapefruit halves with jam and broiling them.
- **Select lean proteins.** Serve poultry, fish, and meatless meals more often. When eating beef, look for leaner cuts (like flank steak, top loin, and sirloin tip), and trim any visible fat before cooking. Small quantities of nut butters (1 to 2 tablespoons), beans, tofu, and eggs make great protein choices.
- **Lovely legumes.** Beans and legumes are nutritious and versatile proteins. You can toss them onto a salad, into a grain dish, and stir them into soups and stews. Replace half the meat in your chili with beans, use bean dip or hummus on sandwiches instead of mayonnaise, make lentil salad instead of pasta salad. Stir black beans into salsa to get a satisfying, heart-healthy, digestive-health promoting dish.

While you're making small changes to the individual food choices you make, remember that what matters most is your overall dietary pattern, which is the total of all the foods you eat. There is no one superfood that will keep you healthy or give you all the energy you need to be active (and one treat will not ruin an otherwise healthful week). Consuming a wide variety of healthful foods is the way to go, provided you achieve the right balance and practice moderation in how much you consume. Beware, however, of ultra-processed foods as these have been found to be health harming (see "Ultra-Processed Foods and Mortality").

NEW FINDING

A Better Burger?

Just because it's plant based doesn't necessarily mean it's a healthier choice (but it might be). Not all plant-based burgers are created equally. Some are highly processed to create animal-product like texture and to "bleed" like burgers (due to additives like beet juice and soy leghemoglobin, a genetically engineered protein). Some contain the same amount of protein as the beef variety, with up to 20 grams of protein in a quarter pound from such sources as peas, soy, beans, and brown rice. Compared to animal-meat burgers, the plant-based varieties generally contain more beneficial fiber. One small study in the *American Journal of Clinical Nutrition* showed plant-based burgers were associated with reductions in low-density lipoprotein (LDL "bad" cholesterol), weight, and trimethylamine-N-oxide (TAMO), a byproduct of red meat metabolism that has been linked with an increased risk of heart attack and stroke. Be sure to read the labels of these plant-based burgers as some contain coconut oil and may have just as much saturated fat as all-beef burgers. Look for plant-based burgers that are made with as few ingredients as possible. Those made from beans may be best, and these can be easily made at home. If you eat fish, it's quick and easy to make a delicious fish patty using canned salmon or tuna. Some have a recipe on the can's label.

American Journal of Clinical Nutrition, Nov. 11, 2020

NEW FINDING

Ultra-Processed Foods and Mortality

Ultra-processed (UPFs) convenience foods are those that are commercially made, typically quite high in sugar and fat, and come packaged in a box, bag, or plastic container. Researchers in Italy wanted to know if these foods might play a role in premature death. Examples of UPFs include fried and salty snacks, ready-to-eat meals, and drinks. UPFs are further defined as those created almost entirely from substances extracted from foods or derived from food constituents with little if any intact foods, and they contain flavors, colors, and other additives that imitate or intensify the sensory qualities of foods (e.g., extra crunchy and vibrantly colored). In search of answers, researchers analyzed data from 22,475 men and women who were followed for eight years. Those who consumed the greatest amount of UPFs were indeed found to have increased risk of death from cardiovascular disease, cerebrovascular disease, and all-cause mortality. The researchers also determined sugar was significantly responsible for the increased risk. Higher consumption of UPFs was associated with consuming more calories overall as well as increased intake of dietary cholesterol and sodium but lower amounts of fiber. Researchers recommend people limit consumption of UPFs and enjoy more natural and minimally processed foods.

American Journal of Clinical Nutrition, Feb. 2, 2021

Planning to Succeed

Research shows that people who plan their meals are more likely to meet recommended dietary guidelines. Before you go to the grocery store, think about what you'll eat during the week, and choose recipes you'd like to make. Make a shopping list to curb impulse buying. Plan to use fresh foods in the days immediately following your shopping trip and cook more pantry- and freezer-based meals (like whole-wheat pasta with cans of beans, tuna, and Italian-seasoned diced tomatoes, or brown rice with frozen edamame and mixed Asian-style vegetables) for meals later in the week.

Batch cooking is a great way to ensure healthy, home-cooked choices when you're short on time. Pick a couple of recipes and schedule a "cooking day," then prep, package, and freeze meals for grab-and-go lunches or quick-defrost ready-made dinners.

Stock your pantry with canned beans and whole grains, fill your freezer with frozen fruits and vegetables, and pull yogurt and fresh veggies to the front of your refrigerator. Planning for healthy choices makes developing new habits much easier (see "Portioning Fruits and Vegetables").

Infusing Flavor

How you cook your food may affect its nutritional value. If you boil vegetables too long, you've dumped nutrients down the drain with the water. If you fry your food in a lot of oil, you've added loads of unnecessary fat and calories to your meal. Instead, try these healthy cooking techniques to get the most nutrition from your healthful food choices:

- **Marinate.** Marinating simply means soaking food in a seasoned liquid before cooking to give it more flavor and to tenderize meat and poultry. A typical marinade blend is one part acid (like vinegar, citrus juice, or wine), two parts oil (like canola), plenty of aromatics and seasonings (like onions, garlic, herbs, and spices), with salt and sugar added to taste. Try ½ cup olive oil; ¼ cup vinegar, lemon juice, or wine; 2 cloves of garlic, crushed; and 2 teaspoons mixed dried herbs. Put all

Portioning Fruits and Vegetables

It's recommended that everyone over 19 years old aim for 1½ to 2 cups of fruit a day and 2½ to 3 cups of vegetables a day. Sometimes it's not so obvious what counts as a "cup."

FRUIT	AMOUNT THAT COUNTS AS 1 CUP OF FRUIT	
apple	• ½ large (3¼" diameter) • 1 small (2¼" diameter)	• 1 cup sliced or chopped
banana	• 1 large (8" to 9")	• 1 cup sliced
cantaloupe	• 1 cup diced or balls	
dried fruit (raisins, prunes, apricots, etc.)	• ½ cup	
100 percent fruit juice	• 1 cup	
grapes	• 1 cup	• 32 seedless
grapefruit	• 1 medium (4" diameter)	• 1 cup sections
mixed fruit (fruit cocktail)	• 1 cup diced or sliced	
orange	• 1 large (3" diameter)	• 1 cup sections
peach	• 1 large (2¾" diameter)	• 1 cup sliced or diced
pear	• 1 medium	• 1 cup sliced or diced
pineapple	• 1 cup chunks, sliced, or crushed	
plum	• 1 cup sliced or diced	• 3 medium or 2 large
strawberries	• 1 cup halved, sliced, or diced	• About 8 large berries
watermelon	• 1 small slice (1" thick)	• 1 cup diced or balls
VEGETABLE	AMOUNT THAT COUNTS AS 1 CUP OF VEGETABLES	
beans and peas	• 1 cup, whole or mashed, cooked	
broccoli	• 1 cup chopped or florets	
cabbage, green	• 1 cup chopped or shredded	
carrots	• 1 cup strips, slices, or chopped • 2 medium	• About 12 baby carrots
cauliflower	• 1 cup pieces or florets	
celery	• 1 cup diced or sliced	• 2 large stalks (11" to 12")
corn	• 1 cup	• 1 large ear (8" to 9")
leafy greens (romaine, watercress, lettuce, endive, escarole)	• 2 cups raw	
peppers (green or red)	• 1 cup chopped	• 1 large pepper (3" diameter, 3¾" long)
potatoes, white	• 1 cup diced or mashed	• 1 medium boiled or baked (2½" to 3" diameter)
pumpkin	• 1 cup mashed, cooked	
spinach	• 1 cup cooked	• 2 cups raw
squash, summer or zucchini	• 1 cup sliced	
squash, winter (acorn, butternut, hubbard)	• 1 cup, cubed, cooked	
tomatoes	• 1 large raw (3")	• 1 cup chopped, canned, or cooked

the ingredients in a gallon sealable bag for easy, no-mess storage and disposal. The thinner or more delicate the food, the less time it should be marinated. Marinate seafood and tofu about 30 minutes; poultry pieces and vegetables, 30 minutes to two hours; and lean meats, 30 minutes to four hours. Use a third to half cup of marinade per pound of food, store food in the refrigerator while marinating, and dispose of the marinade promptly after use.

- **Broil.** Broiling involves cooking food about four to eight inches under the broiler heating element of an oven. You can broil meat, poultry, fish, vegetables, and even fruit. This method works best if you use a slotted broiler pan (or simply use a cooling rack with a cookie sheet underneath). Line the bottom of the pan with aluminum foil for easier cleanup.

- **Poach.** Poaching involves cooking food on the stovetop in a saucepan in barely simmering liquid. Liquid is simmering when small bubbles rise slowly to the liquid's surface. This technique works well for eggs, chicken breast, and firm fish.

- **Roast.** Roasting means cooking food uncovered in the oven, typically without adding liquid. Roasting whole chicken, turkey, and beef is common, but this method works well for fish and vegetables as well. Try drizzling broccoli, cauliflower, or Brussels sprouts with olive oil, sprinkling with salt and pepper (or other seasonings you enjoy), and roasting them to bring out an appealing sweetness.

- **Sauté.** Sautéing involves cooking smaller pieces of food quickly in a little oil in a skillet over medium-high heat, stirring often. Stir-frying is similar but uses high heat and is faster, requiring constant stirring. Sautéing is great for one-pot meals. Brown bite-sized chunks of meat or poultry in a little oil, but don't cook them all the way through. Set the meat aside and put diced, non-leafy veggies

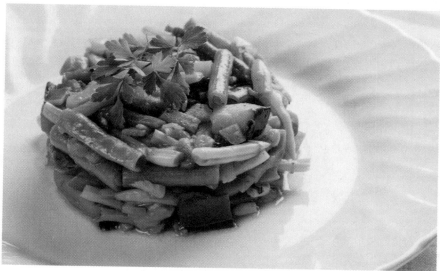

© Angel Luis Simon Martin | Dreamstime

Vegetables cooked in a skillet over medium high heat are particularly satisfying.

in the pan (add onion first and let it soften before adding other vegetables). Add seasoning or sauce, then stir in any greens, and put the meat back into the pan to finish cooking. If you're not starting with raw meat, add pre-cooked meat or beans to warm through near the end of cooking.

- **Steam.** Often used for vegetables, steaming helps retain texture and nutrients. All you need is a saucepan with a lid and a steamer basket that fits in the pot to hold the vegetables out of the boiling water. Steamed vegetables should be "crisp-tender" when finished. Lift the lid occasionally to make sure the veggies are still brightly colored and aren't getting mushy. String beans, peas, sliced or baby carrots, edamame, broccoli, and cauliflower are all delicious steamed.

- **Microwave.** Microwave ovens aren't just good for cooking pre-packaged frozen dinners. They are great for reheating leftovers, quickly defrosting frozen foods, and preparing frozen vegetables. Potatoes and yams can be ready in under 10 minutes in a microwave (just be sure to poke some holes in them first). The next time you're looking for an easy breakfast, crack an egg into the bottom of a glass measuring cup, beat it, cover, and microwave 1 minute. (Grease the cup first

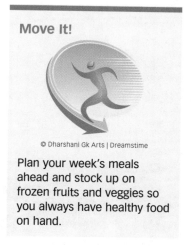

Move It!

© Dharshani Gk Arts | Dreamstime

Plan your week's meals ahead and stock up on frozen fruits and veggies so you always have healthy food on hand.

for easier clean-up.) Toast a whole-grain English muffin and slice some tomato or greens for a quick, power-packed egg sandwich! You can even throw some leftover veggies or protein into the egg before cooking for added flavor and nutrients.

Chef Secrets

Herbs, spices, vinegars, and fruit juices help you cut back on salt, sugar, and fat in dishes while making nutritious foods. A 2018 study published in the *Journal of Food Science* showed that people are more likely to eat more seasoned vegetables and enjoy them more often compared to veggies that are not seasoned.

Herbs come from the leaves of plants (such as basil), while spices may come from the roots (such as ginger), bark (such as cinnamon), berries (such as peppercorns), dried seeds (such as cumin), or flowers/buds of plants (such as saffron and cloves). Compared with herbs, spices typically have stronger flavors, so they're used in smaller amounts.

Carrots are delicious with basil, garlic, thyme, or oregano. Peas work well with tarragon or dill. Dress up green beans with thyme, mint, or tarragon. Try lemon and basil for asparagus, and rosemary and garlic are great with mushrooms. A wide variety of fresh or dried herbs pair well with beef and poultry. Try thyme, coriander, fennel, or rosemary with fish. If you like it hot, red-pepper flakes or a dash of cayenne work with just about

any dish. Don't add too many different flavors at a time. Smelling herbs and spices first may help you decide if they pair well with the dish you're eating.

Vinegars (balsamic, apple cider, white wine, or even plain white) add a mouth-watering bite, but don't overdo it with these strong flavors.

Lemon, lime, and bitter-orange juices added at the end of cooking or squeezed on at the table freshens up fish and vegetables. Try lime and fresh cilantro for a Mexican flair. Low-sodium soy sauce adds an Asian flavor, or experiment with a little fish sauce.

Herbs, spices, aromatics (like onion and garlic), and other flavor enhancers liven up food and add variety and can bring a dose of powerful antioxidant and anti-inflammatory compounds to your plate as well. Experiment by adding small amounts of these flavor enhancers to your foods.

Fortify Your Day

Multiple research studies show that eating breakfast may help prevent or minimize fatigue during exercise and during everyday activities as well. But about 10 percent of Americans don't eat breakfast at all.

Breakfast, like all meals, should follow the MyPlate pattern, but typical American breakfasts—like pancakes with syrup, cereal with milk, and eggs with breakfast meat and buttered bread—rarely do. We've gathered some ideas for plant-based breakfasts that are quick, easy, satisfying, and nutritionally superior to the typical American breakfast fare:

- **For breakfast on the go,** grab a whole-grain snack bar (look for higher fiber and lower sugar), a banana, and a hard-boiled egg or Greek yogurt.
- **Plain yogurt with berries,** granola, and nuts provides fruit, whole grains, protein, and dairy—a power breakfast!
- **Up the protein power** of fashionable avocado toast by layering a sliced

Seasoning will make vegetables extremely appealing.

© Cmillc22 | Dreamstime

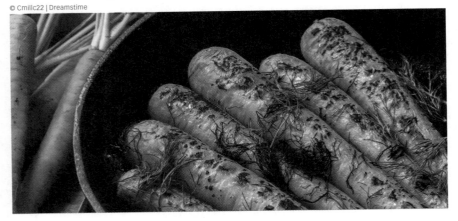

hard-boiled egg with the avocado on whole-grain toast.

- **Spread nut butter** on a whole-grain tortilla and wrap it around a banana. Apple slices, carrots, and celery are great with nut butters too.
- **Eggs are a good** high-protein breakfast choice, but firm tofu can be scrambled with veggies and spices as well. Try either one wrapped in a whole-wheat tortilla and topped with salsa.
- **Cereal.** Tossing a handful of nuts and some fruit into a bowl of cold cereal and milk can help make this choice more healthy, but check the protein, fiber, and added sugars on the cereal-box label. For a warm, filling bowl of hot cereal, choose whole grains like oatmeal over processed cereals like Cream of Wheat or grits. Cooking with low-fat or nonfat milk instead of water adds protein and nutrients, and stirring in finely chopped fruit like apples, dates, or prunes at the start of cooking adds sweetness without the need for added sugars. You could also try a bowl of warm, protein-rich quinoa with fruit and nuts.
- **Think out of the box.** Remember, breakfast doesn't have to be limited to traditional breakfast foods. Nobody says you can't eat leftovers from dinner for breakfast.

An Energizing Lunch

Whether you're eating at the workplace or at home, you'll want a lunch that helps you avoid late-afternoon doldrums. Even in plant-based eating, you can combine protein and whole-grain carbohydrates with fruits and vegetables for extra-energizing nutrients to help you stay satisfied and energized until dinner.

- **Toss the grains and vegetables from dinner with salad greens,** top with rinsed, drained canned beans, and dress. If you're taking lunch to go, bring dressing in a separate container.

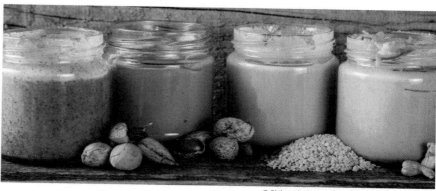

© Oleksandra Naumenko | Dreamstime

- **Sandwich leftover grilled or roasted vegetables** and a slice of cheese and/or some bean dip or hummus between two slices of whole-grain bread or roll it in a whole-grain wrap.
- **Cook, package, and freeze meatless favorites ahead of time,** so you'll have ready-made meals that don't even need an ice pack to stay cold.
- **Try nut butter (like peanut or almond)** on whole-grain bread but use fruit instead of jelly to decrease added sugars and increase flavor and texture. Mashed bananas and apple slices are delicious choices to add.
- **Make a quick bean salad** by tossing beans of your choice with salad dressing. Cut-up veggies and olives make this lunch more delicious and nutritious.
- **Bean-based chili and lentil soups** are great lunch choices, especially during colder weather.

A Purposeful Dinner

When building a healthy evening meal, meatless or not, keep the MyPlate model in mind. Half of your meal should be fruits and vegetables, a quarter should be grain (preferably whole), and a quarter protein. Stews, soups, salads, stir-fries, and even pasta dishes can meet the MyPlate requirements, but keep the proportions in mind. A quarter plate of pasta may look small but toss it with a generous helping of your favorite veggies and some beans or tofu (or poultry or lean meat), and you'll have a sizable,

We are all familiar with peanut butter, but you can also try cashew, almond, and sesame butters.

satisfying meal low in calories and high in energizing, health-promoting nutrients (for helpful suggestions on how to cook small meals for one or two people, see "Cooking for Two").

Top a bowl of cooked whole grains with vegetables and egg, beans, or tofu. Top with sauce or seasonings of your choosing. Try brown rice with seasoned black beans and peppers and add some lettuce or collard greens and a sprinkling of shredded cheese. Or eat quinoa with diced apricots, slivered almonds, and spiced chickpeas. Stewed lentils (like Indian dal) over brown Basmati rice makes a rich and filling meal.

Mix leafy greens (the darker the better) with a variety of colorful vegetables and fruits, and at least one good protein source (like eggs, beans, meat substitute, or tofu, if you're going meatless). To round out the meal, add whole-grain crackers, or warmed whole-wheat pita bread wedges.

If a green salad doesn't sound like dinner, try a taco salad: Start with a quarter of a plate's worth of brown rice and seasoned meatless crumbles, and heap on shredded lettuce and veggies of your choice (such as corn, black olives, and peppers). Top with salsa, and sprinkle with crushed tortilla chips, cilantro, and reduced-fat shredded cheese.

Shredded cabbage tossed with edamame, whole-grain or buckwheat noodles, mandarin oranges, scallions, and peanuts makes a great Asian-style salad. Creamy salad dressings are a big source of bad fats, sodium, and calories. Stick to vinaigrettes and consider shaking up your own.

Make a frittata (an Italian egg-based dish, similar to an omelet or crustless quiche). A typical recipe starts with four eggs and adds ¼ cup of liquid (such as milk, tomato juice, or broth), ¼ teaspoon fresh or dried herbs, and 1 cup of whatever veggies, cheese, pasta, or grains you like. Cook in a hot, well-greased non-stick pan over medium heat for eight to 10 minutes.

It's best to have dinner at a reasonable hour. According to a 2019 study published in *Nutrition, Metabolism & Cardiovascular Diseases,* eating late at night increases LDL ("bad" cholesterol) more than eating the same food earlier in the day, especially if that food is high in fat.

Simple Snacks

A snack can be as simple as a piece of fruit or handful of dry-roasted nuts to tide you over in between meals. If you're looking for snacks with a little more staying power, try combining a whole-food carbohydrate item with a food that provides some protein.

Using the average 2,000-calorie diet as a guide, if meals average 500 calories apiece, that leaves 500 calories for snacks, so keep snacks to 200 to 250 calories or less. See "Satiating Snacks" for nutritious, delicious (meatless) snacks.

With the ways to eat well under our belt, we can now move toward exercise—which may be the most fun part of all.

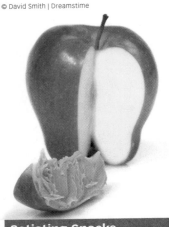

Apple slices with peanut butter give you a healthy snack that combines carbs and protein (and it's a very satisfying choice!).

© David Smith | Dreamstime

Satiating Snacks

Combine an unprocessed carb choice with a protein choice to satisfy hunger better.

CARB CHOICE	+	PROTEIN CHOICE
banana	+	almond butter
celery sticks	+	low-fat spreadable cheese
air-popped popcorn	+	reduced-fat cheese
raisins	+	pistachios
low-sodium tomato juice	+	roasted soy nuts
cucumber slices and carrots	+	hummus
whole-grain crackers	+	reduced-fat cheddar cheese
blackberries	+	hard-boiled egg
apple slices	+	natural, unsweetened peanut butter
berries	+	plain greek yogurt
orange slices	+	part-skim mozzarella cheese sticks
sliced pear	+	light brie cheese
whole-grain melba toast	+	part-skim ricotta cheese
unsweetened dried fruit	+	mixed nuts
dried cranberries	+	pumpkin seeds
halved grapes	+	cottage cheese

Cooking for Two

Cooking for one or two people can be challenging. Fortunately, there are many strategies for shopping and storage that will make preparing healthy meals easier for small households. You can also look for recipes for just two people.

Go to the supermarket with a detailed list based on what you plan to eat that week. Try these shopping strategies:

Bulk Bins. These areas in grocery stores allow you to buy just the amount for you, especailly for grains, legumes, nuts, dried fruits, and many other foods are often available in supermarkets, as well as most health-food stores.

Frozen Section. Frozen fruits and vegetables are at least as nutritious as fresh, if not more so. Choose packages without added salt, fat, or sugars (read the labels!). They will last a long time in the freezer, and they're already cut up, so it saves you prep time and effort.

Small Quantities. Buy a couple of oranges or a few potatoes instead of a bag. It may seem more expensive, but you'll save money in the long run by not throwing out rotten food.

Understand Ripeness. When possible, buy produce in different stages of ripeness. For example, you often can find some ready-to-eat bananas, as well as some green bananas, at the same store. Buying a small amount of each will save you a trip to the supermarket later in the week.

Go to the Salad Bar. For smaller amounts of produce, such as for a minor ingredient of a recipe, check the supermarket salad bar. In some cases, the produce will cost more on the salad bar, but you'll save money in the long run.

Visit the Meat Counter. If you just want one pork chop or chicken breast or a half pound of ground beef, the fresh meat counter is the place to get it.

Include Seafood. Frozen and canned seafood provide easy, healthful protein choices that won't spoil if you can't cook them right away. Look for flavored packets of tuna and salmon for a change from mayonnaise-based preparations.

Freeze It

Use your freezer to store prepped ingredients and save time in the kitchen.

- Label and date home-cooked frozen foods and use them within two to three months for best quality.

- In general, avoid freezing foods that are high in water, such as lettuce and cucumbers. They'll become limp and develop off-flavors and off-colors.

- Cooked potatoes generally don't freeze well, as they tend to become waterlogged and mealy. Thinly sliced potatoes, such as in a casserole, tend to freeze a little better.

- Milk sauces, sour cream, and mayonnaise tend to separate when frozen, and crumb toppings may become soggy.

- Salt loses flavor and can increase rancidity of the fat in frozen meat, so it may be better to wait to add salt until you reheat the meat, if it's needed at all.

- Black pepper, cloves, and garlic tend to become stronger in the freezer. Consider just seasoning dishes lightly with such

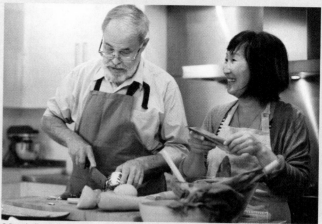
© Rawpixelimages | Dreamstime

When the house gets quiet, and it's just two for dinner, make the preparation as fun as the meal.

flavor enhancers when you make them, then you can add more when reheating or serving.

Do-It-Yourself Entrées. Forget buying pre-made frozen dinners at the supermarket—you can make much healthier options at home. Dishes made with rice, beans, or pasta typically freeze and reheat well, as do meatballs, sliced meatloaf, and leftover roast beef freeze.

Precook and Freeze Chicken Breasts. Many recipes—such as chicken salad, tacos, wraps, and soup—call for precooked boneless, skinless chicken breast meat. Rather than buying salty precooked chicken, cook and freeze your own for later use. One simple method is to put boneless, skinless chicken breasts in a single layer in a baking dish with ¼ to ½ cup water (to prevent the chicken from drying out). Cover and bake in a 350° F oven for 30 to 40 minutes or until completely cooked.

Alternately, you can cook chicken breasts in a slow cooker with ½ cup water on low heat for five to six hours (or eight to nine hours if the chicken is frozen). If you must stack the chicken breasts, be sure to rearrange them once during cooking.

Ready-to-Go Ground Meat. Cook lean ground meat crumbles in one-pound batches and freeze for later use in recipes, such as sloppy Joes, taco salad, or meat sauce for pasta. Cool the ground meat in a shallow container in the refrigerator, then promptly transfer the meat to freezer bags supported by a flat surface, such as a metal pan, until frozen. Once the meat is frozen, you can remove the pan for more efficient stacking.

Freeze Whole Grains. Brown rice, whole wheat berries (including ancient varieties such as farro and Kamut), oat groats, and other intact whole grains—ones that haven't been ground into flour or flaked—take longer to cook. Cook extra and freeze (or refrigerate) them for later use. They can be used in soups, stews, casseroles, salads, pilafs, or simply as hot cereal.

Watch portions along with food choices, plan, don't be afraid to try new things, and remember that eating healthy food should be delicious and satisfying—not a sacrifice.

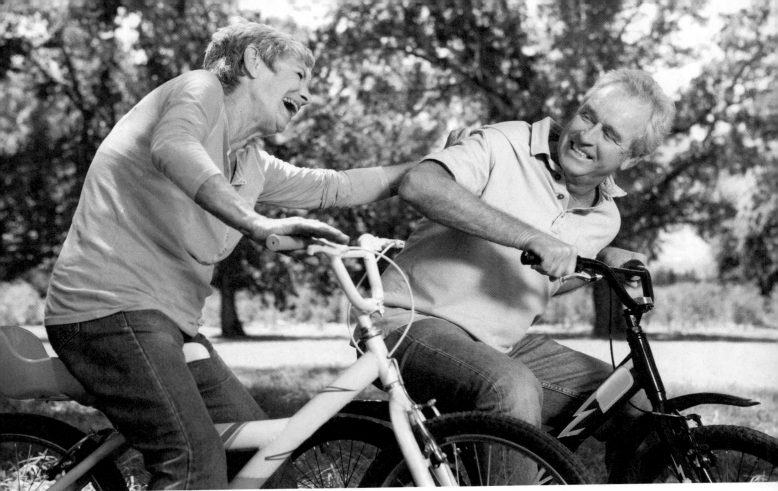

Regular activity is good for your mind, body, and spirit.

7 Exercise Improves Life

If you are willing to build the exercise habit, your whole life can transform, no matter how old or deconditioned you are right now. You might need a little help to get started, and it might take some willpower. But sticking with a program bestows a sense of confidence, purpose, and courage in having done something out of your comfort zone. Taking just one more step, another lap in the pool, or lifting a barbell just one more time when you think you can't is incredibly satisfying. Just try it and see what happens.

Exercise makes just about every aspect of life and living better. Science validates that statement in many studies. For example, exercise has been shown to reduce inflammation in the brain and the body, which may help protect against many chronic diseases as well as cognitive conditions. In a 2019 study of sedentary but otherwise healthy older adults (ages 60 through 88), published in *Applied Physiology, Nutrition and Metabolism,* researchers found that a vigorous form of exercise called HIIT (high-intensity interval training) was particularly beneficial for improving high-interference memory. This type of memory helps us distinguish fine details, such as the differences among one car from another car of the same make or model. Research has also shown that improvements in fitness correlate with improvements in memory. And that's just the tip of of the iceberg of what exercise can do for you. Moderate-intensity exercise, like jogging or cycling, releases natural endocannabinoids (the same as those derived from cannabis/marijuana), which can relieve pain and make you feel happier.

Move It!

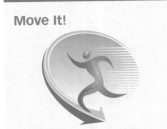

Your immune system gets a slight boost from every little bit of exercise you do. Consistent, regular exercise is best, but never give up. Do what you can!

Exercise Immunology

The field of investigation known as "exercise immunology" emerged some 20 years ago. Studies have shown that flexing skeletal muscles stimulates molecules that commune with immune cells throughout the body.

The immune system especially benefits from cardiovascular exercise that utilizes whole-body, large muscle groups by releasing white blood cells (WBCs) into circulation between the blood and tissues for constant monitoring for antigens (see "What Is an Antigen?"). More specifically, the released neutrophil concentrations, which are considered the first responders to microbial infections, increase during and after exercise. According to the American College of Sports Medicine, WBC concentrations can increase within the first 10 minutes of aerobic and resistance exercise.

Lowering Inflammation

According to a review study published in the May 2019 issue of the *Journal of Sport and Health Science*, when repeated on a regular basis, multiple benefits are realized from moderate exercise, including decreased incidences of illness and dampened systemic inflammation. A review study bases its findings on numerous existing studies with defined parameters for inclusion. In this case, the review analyzed 179 studies and consolidated the findings in the publication.

One of the studies analyzed included 1,000 adults ages 18 to 85; 60 percent were female and 40 were male. Two groups (sedentary people versus exercisers) were compared over a 12-week period. The exercise group engaged in at least 20 minutes of aerobic exercise, on average five days per week. The researchers found that exercise frequency was associated with a reduced number of days with upper respiratory tract infections (URTI). The number of days with URTI was 43 percent lower in those who exercised at least five days per week. Despite that intense exercise

bouts can increase some inflammatory compounds immediately after exercise, there is evidence that exercise decreases overall inflammation in the body. Also, physically fit people have lower levels of inflammatory biomarkers when they are at rest compared to people who are obese and unfit. Persistent, or chronic, inflammation is linked with many disorders, including arthritis, atherosclerosis, cardiovascular disease, kidney disease, type 2 diabetes, obesity, osteoporosis, dementia, depression, and some cancers.

Counteracting Age-Related Immune Change

Everything changes with age, some for the good, some not so much. Many people become wiser and more patient with age. The immune system, however, is known to be less efficient through time.

What Is an Antigen?

An antigen is any substance (e.g., bacteria, viruses, pollen) that triggers your immune system to produce antibodies against it. The resulting antibodies convey that your immune system does not recognize the substance and is trying to neutralize it to prevent spread. Disease-specific antibodies have been found in blood samples of people who had COVID-19, meaning they had the disease and their immune systems had formed a response.

Immune System

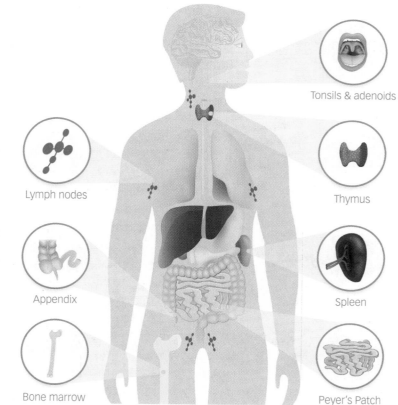

Lymph nodes

Appendix

Bone marrow

Tonsils & adenoids

Thymus

Spleen

Peyer's Patch

© Designua | Dreamstime

Your immune system protects you. Healthy food and exercise help keep it going strong.

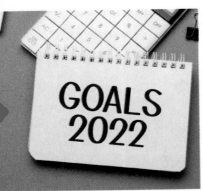

© Andrei ASKIRKA | Dreamstime

Experts typically advocate for SMART goals: Specific, Measurable, Achievable, Realistic, Time-bound. This can help you accomplish goals year after year.

The term "immune senescence" refers to the age-related decline of the immune system, which results in increased susceptibility to infections, diseases, and neurologic disorders. Healing also takes more time. But it doesn't necessarily have to be a steady downward decline. Studies have shown that even later in life, you can influence how your immune system responds to challenges. And exercise is a significant contributor.

An older study that is still referenced today compared 30 sedentary elderly women to highly conditioned elderly women who made choices such as participating in state and national senior games and endurance races. It showed that the conditioned women had higher levels of natural killer cells and better T-lymphocyte (T cells) function. T cells are major immune system players. The conditioned women also showed reduced rates of illness compared to their sedentary counterparts.

In addition, data shows that a regular exercise habit can improve vaccination response, lower circulatory levels of inflammatory cells, and lengthen telomeres (the end caps of DNA which, when shortened, accelerate age-related demise).

On the flip side, people with sarcopenia (age-related loss of muscle) take longer to heal after infections and surgery. People with severely weakened muscles have double the risk for infection after surgery.

But all is not lost even if you haven't seen the inside of a gym for a very long time. Positive immune responses from exercise occur within a single session. Although, for sustained improvement, you need to be active most days a week. Make it a goal to exercise a minimum five days/week doing at least 30 minutes of moderate intensity aerobic exercise (walking, biking, etc.). If you are just starting out, try two to three 10- to 15-minute walks throughout the day and gradually build the walking duration until you reach 30 minutes. Take breaks as needed.

Prove It to Yourself

If exercise constantly falls to the bottom of your to-do list, run your own personal research study. Define a length of time, for example 21 days, where you will make exercise a priority. Your study needs a goal (e.g., I will walk every day for 30 minutes, I will take three Pilates classes per week, I will train for a 5K, I will earn a yoga-teacher certification). Whatever it is, schedule it into your day, know what you are going to do, and for how long.

Your study also needs an objective. What is it you're trying to prove? Of course, it must be within the realm of possibility (personal trainers can help with this). For example, if you want to see how exercise impacts your stress level, use a simple scale, defining 1 as no stress to 5 as extreme stress. Log those numbers before and after each exercise session and see what happens after a few weeks. Similarly, you can set a strength, distance, flexibility, or balance objective. Again, it all should be designed to be realistic, yet challenging.

Signing up for a class or competition, especially if it's a group effort, can help strengthen your resolve and get you out the door.

Set Up for Success

For most people, fitness as a lifestyle requires making some changes to daily routines and habits. Behavior change can be challenging, but science offers proven ideas that help many people. In a short time, you'll reap the benefits of physical activity, and that can motivate you to stay the course.

Create the Habit. Getting into the exercise habit doesn't happen overnight. Studies suggest it may take about 10 weeks of consistently repeating a desired behavior, such as fitness walking, to form a new habit. The more consistently you exercise, the easier it should get and the more likely it will become a habit. At that point, skipping it will feel strange.

Anchor It. You are more likely to exercise if you make it a regular part of your day and anchor it to an existing habit, just as you might do for brushing your teeth before you go to bed. To anchor exercise to an existing habit, think about what time of day you'd like to exercise. For example, if you'd like to go for a walk in the evening after dinner, you might anchor your habit like this: After I do the dishes, I will go for a walk.

Find a Buddy. Many people find it motivating (and more fun!) if they exercise with someone else or check into walking groups through senior centers or nature centers. Consider asking a friend, family member, coworker, or neighbor if they'd like to join you for a walk, hike, or a trip to the fitness center. You also can get peer support from virtual exercise communities using smartphone apps and websites, and many organizations can help you find a group to exercise with in person.

Choose Fun. No matter what type of exercise you're doing, it's important to select activities you enjoy. Trying something new can boost motivation and having fun increases the odds you'll do it again.

In one study, women who were asked to use a hula hoop for 30 minutes reported that they had significantly higher intentions of doing aerobic exercise in the next month compared with those who had walked on a treadmill for 30 minutes.

Maybe you've always wanted to try ballroom dancing or tap, or maybe there's a local adult recreation league for the sport you played in school. Join a bowling league, start a walking book club, try a yoga class, or see how it feels to hit a punching bag.

Set Goals and Track Progress. Setting clear, manageable goals can be motivational, and tracking your activity can help you assess your progress toward those goals. Record how much weight you lifted, the number of sets and reps, steps taken, distances run, or exercise classes attended. Seeing tangible levels of improvement may encourage you to keep going, and a lack of improvement could signal the need to change your approach.

Missing a single day of exercise won't necessarily derail your exercise habit, but missing a whole week could. Aim to be as consistent in your routine as you can, but don't beat yourself up if you get off track. Every day is a new day to try to do a little bit better.

Movement Opportunities

Whether you choose to exercise at home; go to a local park, pool, or community center; join a Y or health club; or even hire a personal trainer, there is no wrong way to be physically active.

You may enjoy the social aspect often found with joining a local gym. Feeling connected to a community of others is a valuable benefit of exercise. Whether you're running your first 5K, taking yoga classes, or entering a gym for the first time in years, there are other people doing the same thing, and it doesn't take long for friendships to form (see "Finding a Gym or Fitness Club").

Remind yourself that it can be challenging to fit in exercise. Some people find that exercising in the morning before they get too busy works best. Others prefer to exercise in the late afternoon to unwind and de-stress.

If you don't have 30 minutes to exercise, schedule exercise in 10-minute sessions during the day, such as morning, lunchtime, and as an afternoon break.

Finding a Gym or Fitness Club

Gyms, health clubs, and boutique studios (e.g., for yoga, Pilates, cycling) house fitness equipment and exercise classes under one roof and provide an opportunity to socialize with others interested in physical activity. The local Y is a great resource in many areas. You also can go to gymsandfitnessclubs.com and put in your zip code to find clubs in your area.

Your insurance plan may qualify you for a discount at certain health clubs. The SilverSneakers program offers unlimited access to more than 14,000 participating gyms and fitness centers to people on Medicare. Visit the website silversneakers.com or call 866-584-7389 to find out more.

Conversely, if you can prove you go to a gym or health club regularly, you may qualify for a discount or incentive bonus on your health insurance. Before you choose a health-insurance plan or gym based on discounts, check which gyms in your area are included in the discount offer, and visit them to make sure they're a facility you'd want to join. Our checklist gives you ideas on what to look for and, if comparing facilities, you can use the list to help decide which you prefer.

Gym Assessment Checklist		
QUESTION	YES	NO
Did the gym offer you a tour when you visited?		
Were there friendly members your age working out at the gym?		
Is the staff experienced with older adults?		
Are the personal trainers accredited for senior-fitness training?		
Does the staff routinely interact with customers?		
Are personal training sessions available?		
Are there exercise classes appropriate for your age and fitness level?		
Is the equipment easy to adjust, such as seat height?		
Does the resistance equipment use compressed air (pneumatic) resistance? (Pneumatic equipment is easier to adjust with a push of a button than weight stacks.)		
Do the weight settings have a large variance, so you can start small and work up?		
Is there a trial membership available (free or very low cost)?		
Is there a membership discount for seniors?		
Are there start-up fees, monthly fees, policies for suspending membership temporarily, and membership-cancellation policies?		
Is the parking lot adequate and safely well lit?		
Are the rooms sanitized and clean?		

The latest physical activity guidelines say that there is no minimum amount of time you need to reach in a single session to make activity valuable.

Regardless of when you plan to exercise, treat exercise like an appointment that you must keep. Schedule it on a calendar, daily planner, smartphone, or wherever you keep your appointments.

Home Gyms

You don't need to leave home to get active. You can get your heart rate up at home by just getting chores done. Cleaning and yardwork can get your blood pumping. Or you can walk up and down the stairs, dance during television commercials, use cans or milk jugs as weights, or follow an exercise video or DVD. If you have a video-game system, many excellent games are designed to give you a workout, from dance games to virtual personal trainers.

For some people, buying fitness equipment for home use may be a good alternative to joining a gym, especially if it makes it more likely you'll exercise (you don't have to get in the car and go somewhere). You can purchase low-cost stability balls, free weights (dumbbells), and resistance bands, as well as pricier equipment, such as home weight machines and cardiovascular workout equipment, such as treadmills and exercise bikes.

Some businesses rent exercise equipment, such as treadmills, rowers, elliptical machines, and weight equipment. Renting gives you a chance to try machines and determine how much you'd really use them. It also may be handy for temporary locations, such as a winter home. Joining a gym, however, most likely would be a lot more budget friendly.

If you already have an outdoor bicycle, consider buying a bike-trainer device, which allows you to ride your regular bike in place indoors. You'll pay a fraction of the cost compared to a dedicated exercise bike.

Especially for larger purchases, be sure to try exercise equipment before you buy it. If you've never used an elliptical machine, for example, don't buy one simply because your friend raves about hers. Stores typically have floor models you can try. To save money, check stores that sell second-hand exercise equipment. If you're tired of the equipment you have and want something different, some exercise equipment stores pay cash for used equipment, although you may be able to make more money selling it on your own.

Creative Options

Getting outside your home can shake up your routine and might make exercising more interesting and fun, but that doesn't mean you have to join a gym or a health club. Walking, jogging, biking, golfing, bowling, playing basketball, or joining a softball team or biking club are all great ways to increase activity and improve your health. Other ideas for making the most of opportunities right outside your door. For example:

- **Shopping malls** are a great place to walk in all weather.
- **Large community spaces,** such as parks, zoos, and museums, provide space for walking.
- **Faith-based organizations** and churches sometimes offer exercise programs.
- **Hospital-sponsored wellness and rehabilitation centers** employ physical therapists and other experts to assist with recovery from injury and illness.
- **Parks and recreation departments** can provide information about indoor and outdoor activities, bike/walking trails, public swimming pools, and more.
- **The StrongWomen Initiative,** founded by Miriam Nelson, PhD, at Tufts University, targets women in midlife and older. StrongWomen programs include strength training and heart-disease prevention (aerobic activity) programs and are offered in at least

29 states. Visit strongwomen.org to learn more.

- **Active.com,** an event registration website, helps you find physical activity events in your area, such as 5K races (walk or run), bicycling group events, and marathons. A related site, activeendurance.com, provides resources for helping organize a fun run and other race events.

Hiring a Coach

Professional athletes have coaches, perhaps you should get one, too. A personal trainer can provide the one-on-one attention to help you get where you want to go. A personal trainer should assess your health and fitness level, design a program that meets your individual needs, teach you how to perform exercises safely, and motivate you to reach for a higher level of fitness. They are available at many health clubs and Ys, but there are also some who operate private businesses, offering training in storefronts or right in your own home. Personal trainers are typically paid by the hour.

Look for a personal trainer who is certified by a nationally recognized organization that is reputable, such as the American College of Sports Medicine or the National Strength and Conditioning Association, and who has a four-year degree in exercise science, kinesiology, physical education, or a related health-and-fitness field.

You should be aware that some personal trainers offer nutrition counseling, but very few are trained nutrition professionals. Always be sure to ask about their training. Your health-care provider can recommend a nutritionist.

Track Your Progress

Tracking your physical activity can help you see your progress, stay focused on your goals, and keep you motivated to continue. One research study provides evidence that using an activity tracker can help with reaching weight-loss goals. The subjects in the study (mostly middle-aged women) lost more weight when activity trackers were added to their weight-loss programs.

Simple Logging

If you prefer low-tech methods, you can use a notebook to record your progress. For aerobic exercise, record the date, activity, minutes, and distance. For resistance, record the date and each exercise with sets, reps, and weight lifted. You can use these records to see how far you've come over time and plan your next step.

Activity-Tracking Gadgets

Numerous step counters, activity trackers, fitness wristbands, and other gadgets are available to help monitor you during exercise, track physical activity, and help keep you motivated to move your body. Sophisticated devices such as heart-rate monitors are available, too. In general, the best choice is whatever accurately gives you the information you need, is easy to use, and fits your budget.

An article published in the *Journal of Sports Medicine* (2018) found 25 high-quality studies that addressed the efficacy of wearable activity devices used in a comprehensive weight-loss program. While not much benefit was seen in young adults, the study found middle age or older people lost more weight when activity trackers were added to short-term weight-loss interventions.

Step Trackers. If you walk, run, or jog, a pedometer can help you track your distance in terms of steps. One mile is about 2,000 steps, depending on your stride. Pedometers are small step-counting devices that can be strapped to your waistband or fit in your pocket and generally range in price from $20 to $50. Various smartphone apps are also available to track the number of steps and distance covered.

When Inclement Weather or "Life" Interrupts

If your activity of choice is done outside, bad weather can put a real damper on your exercise plans. That's when you go to Plan B. Indoor exercise provides a great alternative for staying active year-round. Options include:

- Use a home-exercise video.
- Clean your house with vigorous activities such as mopping and vacuuming.
- Buy your own exercise equipment.
- Walk at a local mall or similar large public facility.
- Go to a local recreation center or community center.
- Go to a gym or health club. Some offer day passes so you may not have to commit to a long-term membership.

If you must take a break from exercise because you're sick or injured, as soon as you're able, pick up exercise again. Start at a lower level than where you left off, and gradually work back up to the level of intensity you were previously doing.

Admittedly, when traveling or during holidays, it is challenging to exercise. It helps to set up your environment to support activity. For example, choose a hotel with a swimming pool or a fitness room and pack your exercise clothes or swimsuit. Alternately, take along an exercise DVD that you can play on your laptop computer. There are also online exercise videos you can view.

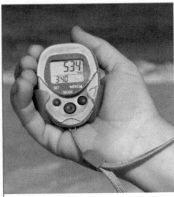

© Angela Schmidt | Dreamstime

Most smartphones have fitness apps, but a simple pedometer can help you just track your steps.

Daily Steps Value

NUMBER OF STEPS	ACTIVITY LEVEL
0–4,999	sedentary
5,000–7,499	low active
7,500–9,999	somewhat active
10,000–12,500	active
12,500 or more	highly active

If your goal is to decrease how sedentary you are throughout the day and walk more, you can use a pedometer to monitor your physical activity. Some people aim for 10,000 steps a day (which is about five miles), but that number may be too high or too low for you. You may want to wear the pedometer for several days to get your baseline before setting a steps-per-day goal. See "Daily Steps Value" for a general guide to classifying your activity level based on step counts.

To test the accuracy of a pedometer, attach it to your belt or waistband on either side of the front of your body so that it's in line with the center of your kneecap and walk 50 steps at your typical walking pace. If it reads between 47 and 53 steps, it's likely reasonably accurate and your placement is good.

If the reading varies more than three steps above or below 50, reposition it on your waistband and repeat the test (try the opposite side of your waist, if necessary, too).

If your waistband is loose, that can lead to undercounting steps. If no position is accurate, the device itself may not be good and you may need to return it for a refund.

Keep in mind that most pedometers are fairly accurate at speeds of 2.5 mph and above; however, even some of the most accurate pedometers miscount steps at slower speeds, according to the American College of Sports Medicine.

If you carry your smartphone with you wherever you go, including during exercise, then a pedometer app may work well for you. A study that compared the accuracy of dedicated fitness trackers versus smartphone fitness apps for counting steps suggests smartphone apps can be a good choice.

If you walk or run for exercise and want to know more than just how many steps you've taken, there are countless free- or low-cost activity smartphone apps, which you can locate by checking the health and fitness category at your app store. Many allow you to track food intake as well as activity if you're trying to lose weight or eat healthier. Some even have built-in support groups.

Digital Bands and Watches. Many of these products track everything from steps, heart rate, and calories to sleep patterns, and some can even automatically recognize when you are performing some types of exercise. Some have screens that display data, while others require a smartphone to view your information. The latest high-end smartwatches have music storage and allow you to check messages, get calendar alerts, and even make purchases right from your watch.

Most of these products are meant to be worn around the clock, and some measure your quality of sleep. Most come with interchangeable bands to go with your style for the day.

Prices may range from $60 to well over $200. Such fitness bands typically have memory and download options, so you can store your physical activity data or share it on social networking sites, if you would like to do so.

Choose a fitness tracker that fits your budget and your needs. If you swim, for example, a waterproof model would be the best choice. Because technology changes quickly, check for the latest reviews on whatever smartphone app, fitness band, smartwatch, or other device you are considering purchasing.

Heart-Rate Monitors. Heart rate is a measure of how fast your heart is beating. Measuring beats per minute during exercise is a shortcut to gauging exercise intensity. If your heart rate goes over your target, you'll know it's time to slow down, and seeing it below the target rate can motivate you to work a little harder (see "Assessing Exertion").

A heart-rate monitor helps you keep tabs on your exercise intensity without the need to stop and take your pulse. These devices are available as chest straps, arm bands, or even earphones that track your workouts while you listen to music. Many fitness trackers and smartwatches include heart-rate monitors, so you may not need a second device if you choose to use one of these devices.

The latest models do more than just monitor heart rate. Features include counting reps during strength training, tracking your run, and sending data to smartphone apps. There are a variety of features and types of monitors on the market (including some better suited to cycling and waterproof models for swimmers), so choose the monitor best suited to your needs.

Athletic Wear

While expensive clothing is not needed for exercise, whatever you wear should be comfortable and allow for easy movement. Clothing and socks that wick moisture can help if you sweat a lot. Shoes should be comfortable and supportive.

Shoes should provide cushioning to help protect against muscle and joint injuries. Replace athletic shoes after three to six months of regular use or when you've put approximately 350 to 500 miles of walking or running on them. If you're not sure how long you've had your shoes or how many miles are on them, replace shoes when the tread is worn out or your feet feel tired after exercising. People who have reduced sensation in their feet (a possible complication of diabetes) need to pay attention to their shoes and should talk to a foot-care expert before beginning an exercise program. If you're not sure you're using the right shoes for exercise, go to a shoe store that specializes in athletic shoes for expert help choosing the right shoe for you.

Assessing Exertion

Use the talk test: If you can carry on a conversation without any difficulty, you may be exercising below your target zone. If you can carry on a conversation but need to stop speaking now and then to catch your breath, you probably are in your target heart rate zone. If talking is difficult or impossible, you may be overdoing it and may need to ease up a bit.

You can determine how hard you are working by measuring your heart rate—the number of times your heart beats in one minute. Many smartwatches can do this for you.

To get the most benefit from aerobic exercise, you should exercise hard enough and long enough to get your heart rate into the target range for your age. See below for an estimate of the numbers you should be trying to reach.

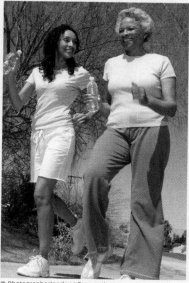
© Photographerlondon | Dreamstime

Walking with a friend is great fun, and it gives you a natural way to do the "talk test."

Heart Rate Targets

If you're just beginning an exercise program, aim for the lower end of the target zone. As you become more fit, increase the intensity of your exercise by aiming for a higher target heart rate. Remember, even the most vigorous exercise is performed below your estimated maximum heart rate. Certain blood pressure medications, sometimes called beta-blockers, can lower heart-rate recommendations. Check with your doctor if you are on blood-pressure medications, or if you have a pacemaker or irregular heart rhythm.

Estimated Heart Rate by Age* in beats per minute (bpm)

	MAXIMUM HEART RATE	MODERATE	VIGOROUS**
Age	220 minus your age in years	Target = 50–70 Percent of Maximum	Target = 70–85 Percent of Maximum
20	200	100–140	140–170
25	195	98–137	137–166
30	190	95–133	133–162
35	185	93–130	130–157
40	180	90–126	126–153
45	175	88–122	122–149
50	170	85–119	119–144
55	165	82–115	115–140
60	160	80–112	112–136
65	155	77–108	108–132
70	150	75–105	105–127
75	145	72–101	101–123
80	140	70–98	98–119
85	135	67–94	94–115

*This chart provides estimates of maximum and target heart rates by age using one formula. This is a guide, not a recommendation. Online calculators (such as active.com/fitness/calculators/heartrate), your doctor, or a fitness expert may use slightly different ranges. **Do not exercise at maximum heart rate. Maintaining heart rate above 85 percent for prolonged periods can put excessive strain on your heart and circulatory system.

Dressing for Cold

If you plan to exercise outside, dress in layers so you can shed a layer as you warm up during exercise. If you plan to exercise outdoors in the early morning or evening when lighting is dim, wear bright or reflective clothing. If it's raining or snowing, wear a waterproof coat or jacket.

If it is cold outside, wear several layers of loose clothing: Overly tight clothing can keep your blood from flowing freely and lead to loss of body heat, and the space between the layers traps warm air. Cover your extremities with a hat, scarf, and gloves. Warm up your muscles before you go outside.

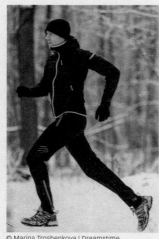

© Marina Troshenkova | Dreamstime

In cold weather, wear breathable, warm clothing that allows moisture to evaporate. A hat and gloves are also wise to wear.

⬧ **Shop at the end of the day,** which is when your feet are at their largest.
⬧ **Measure your feet each time you buy shoes.** Foot sizes change with age.
⬧ **Wear the same thickness of socks** you intend to wear during exercise.
⬧ **Select shoes that are made for the exercise you plan to do,** such as walking, running, or cycling (yes, it matters).
⬧ **The sole should be shock-absorbing and non-skid.** To check this, press on the sole to make sure it has some give and walk in the shoes.
⬧ **The shoe should bend at the ball of your foot** (the space between your toes and arch), not in the middle of the shoe.
⬧ **The shoe should be comfortable when you try it on.** Break-in periods are a thing of the past.
⬧ **Choose shoes with a wide toe box,** so you can wiggle your toes inside the shoe and your feet have room to spread out normally when you step down.
⬧ **Check that the shoe is long enough**—a thumb's width between your big toe and the front of the shoe.
⬧ **Be sure the insole of the shoe molds to the shape of your foot.** The arch shouldn't be too high or too low.
⬧ **The shoe material should allow your foot to breathe,** such as via an open weave on the top of the shoe.
⬧ **When you walk,** the heel shouldn't slip.

Dedicated exercise attire is useful in many classes and exercise disciplines. In Pilates and yoga classes, form-fitting clothing prevents snags in equipment or shirts from falling forward during certain exercises. Dance fitness classes require the right shoes as does playing golf and bowling. The right clothes also can help provide motivation and dedication. Athletic pants allow more flexion than jeans in running sports. Just slipping on the shoes, shirt, and pants for class can help you get in the mood.

A Word on Supplements

Supplements and specialty sports foods, such as nutrition bars, energy gels, and protein shakes, are promoted to active people and athletes—and they're big business, with billions of dollars in annual sales.

Unless you're an endurance athlete spending more than 60 to 90 minutes in exercise daily or competing in long-distance events, you most likely don't need specialty sports products.

Many gyms and nutrition stores, as well as supermarkets, sell protein powder supplements that can be mixed into water, juice, milk, smoothies, or other beverages. Most physically active people easily can meet their protein needs with food. If you choose to use protein supplements, watch for added sugars, and remember that the body can only use so much protein—any extra is broken down for energy, and excesses can be stored as fat (see "Why You 'Hit the Wall'").

Why You "Hit the Wall"

You have limited carbohydrate stores for exercise in the form of glycogen stored in your liver and muscles, and once you run out you either must decrease your exercise intensity or stop altogether. This is what's called "hitting the wall" during endurance exercise—the sudden fatigue and loss of energy when your carbohydrate stores fall short.

Endurance activities like marathon running or long-distance cycling are more likely to lead to carbohydrate shortfalls, and those who participate in such activities may consume carbohydrates during exercise to prevent an energy shortage. Carbohydrates that enter the bloodstream quickly are ideal for this purpose.

Avoid foods with fat or fiber, which slow down the release of sugars into the bloodstream. Sports gels, energy chews, gummies, and sports drinks will help, but a healthy small box of raisins may work just as well.

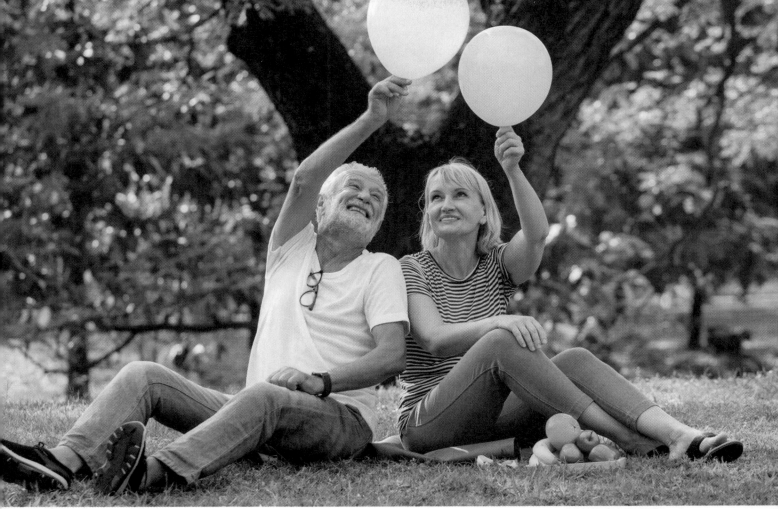

Put together some simple healthy foods and go outside and play.

8 Make the "Golden" Years Fun

This chapter continues to make the case that a healthy, balanced lifestyle can make senior years truly golden years. Research shows how profoundly exercise stimulates well-being in mind and body, and how nourishing your body with healthy foods influences everything from head to toe.

Staying the course for the long run is among the most challenging aspects of embarking on lifestyle changes. That's true whether you have a chronic condition or not. If you're completely out of shape, know that exercise can help you become more mobile even if you're well into your senior years, and studies support that conclusion.

Researchers at the Jean Mayer USDA Human Nutrition Research Center on Aging at Tufts published a small study in 2019 in the *Journals of Gerontology Medical Sciences* that compared what happens when two groups of deconditioned 80-year-old women received either health education counseling or group-based physical activity. You can likely guess the outcome. But one detail is particularly noteworthy—those who participated in exercise at least once per week had meaningful improvements.

So, it's possible to improve health and well-being even if you're deconditioned at 80 years of age. If just once a week can make some difference, imagine what might happen if you devoted five days per week to intentional movement. A 2019 study published in *Restorative Neurology and Neuroscience* found that people with rheumatoid arthritis experienced decreased inflammation

Move It!

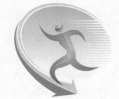

Exercise helps you age better in so many ways. It can reduce fall risk, keep your immune system stronger, and help you maintain an independent lifestyle.

Exercise Enhances Thinking and Memory

Physical activity can improve thinking and memory even if you haven't worked out in a long time, according to a new study involving adults ages 55 and older. Researchers discovered that previously unconnected portions of the brain became more connected and more flexible as study participants started to move more regularly. Specifically, the study found that aerobic exercise had a positive influence on the medial temporal lobe (MTL) network, one of the earliest brain regions to be affected by Alzheimer's disease. The study tested the effect of a 20-week twice-weekly dance-based aerobic exercise intervention and compared outcomes to a non-exercise group.

All participants received extensive cognitive tests, fitness, lifestyle assessments, and an invitation to undergo functional magnetic resonance brain scans. Participants were African Americans, average age 65, with a mean educational level of 14 years and included men and women. Exercise exertion was at moderate intensity. Researchers concluded that exercise exerts both rehabilitative and protective effects upon MTL function that were not observed in the control group. Moreover, exercise participants improved their ability to learn and retain information as well as to apply knowledge in new situations.

According to the researchers, this kind of thinking tends to diminish with age, but the exercisers achieved higher test scores compared to when they started the study. Researchers also suggest that the social connectivity aspect of a group exercise class may have also influenced the outcomes.

Neurobiology of Learning and Memory, January 2021

and improved functional status with 120 minutes of yoga per day, five days per week. Yes, that's two hours per day, but yoga involves resting, conscious breathing exercises as well as stretching, balancing and flowing movement.

And keep in mind that, according to the National Institutes of Health, most benefits from exercise are gained with at least 150 to 300 minutes of moderate physical activity per week. That's just a half hour to an hour five days per week.

Energize Your Life

A lack of energy, difficulty sleeping, and losing zest for life are some of the complaints voiced by people as they age. It is true that the body's overall metabolism slows with each passing decade. We lose muscle mass and gain more fat. That's why food choices and physical activity become even more important. Daily choices can mean the difference between feeling energized or fatigued and being fit or fat. A study published in the *Annals of Internal Medicine* (2017) showed that high sedentary time (12.5 or more hours daily) is associated with a greater risk of premature death.

Research shows that nearly 90 percent of older adults in the United States watch television on a given day, at an average of nearly five hours daily. Maybe television isn't such a lure for you, but perhaps computer time, reading, or some other sedentary activity is. Regardless of what you're doing (or not doing!), it's important to get up and get moving frequently throughout the day.

It seems counterintuitive, but exercise boosts energy. As the circulatory system is stimulated, more blood flows throughout the body and into the brain—energizing both with richly oxygenated blood. And that's not all: A study in *Mayo Clinic Proceedings* (2019) found that exercise can reduce health-harming visceral fat, that deep layer of fat that surrounds organs and increases disease risk.

You might think that exercise won't matter that much as you get older, but that's incorrect. Not only can it improve how you feel physically, it benefits your brain even if you haven't worked out in a long time (see "Exercise Enhances Thinking and Memory").

If you've been inactive for a while, start at a low level of activity and work your way up slowly over time. Some older adults avoid exercise and physical activity due to fear of injury, but the risks of being sedentary are far greater than any that might come with starting light activity. Your local National Association of Area Agencies on Aging headquarters (n4a.org) may assist you in finding a physical activity program for older adults.

Remember that the social support of walking groups can help older adults increase physical activity, as well as improve health. That's why many church groups and senior-living centers offer exercise programs, such as classes on tai chi, yoga, and tap dancing. A strong core (the trunk of your body) can also help you sit, stand, and move with better posture and balance.

Nourishing Body and Mind

As you age, you need fewer calories but more vitamins and minerals. That is because the absorption of nutrients in the digestive tract becomes less efficient, increasing requirements for certain nutrients as you age. So, focus on eating more nutrient-dense foods. For easy tips see "Calorie and Nutrient Needs."

According to the National Council on Aging, 16 percent of independent older adults are at high risk for malnutrition due to their dietary choices. Research shows that community-dwelling older adults in Western countries are prone to a low dietary intake of vitamin D, thiamin, riboflavin, calcium, magnesium, and selenium.

Older adults often consume too little protein for muscle strength and have low levels of vitamin B_{12} (important to prevent neurological deterioration and for red blood cells) and vitamin D (essential for calcium absorption). They may also be iron-deficient.

Focus on eating the most nutrient-rich foods you can to meet your nutritional needs and remain within your calorie limit. Avoid empty calories. Nutrient deficiencies can impact both your health and your quality of life but eating well can ensure you get everything you need.

Tufts' MyPlate for Older Adults

The easiest way to ensure you are getting the nutrients you need is to follow a healthy dietary pattern. Tufts' MyPlate for Older Adults is like the

Calorie and Nutrient Needs

These healthy strategies can help increase calories (if needed), protein, and nutrition:

- Make sure foods high in protein are consumed at all meals.
- Add 1 to 4 tablespoons dry milk powder to liquid milk, smoothies, mashed potatoes, casseroles, and hot or cold cereals.
- Enjoy whole milk and yogurt rather than skim or low-fat.
- Add grated cheese to eggs, pasta, vegetables, soups, salads, and casseroles.
- Sprinkle wheat germ, nuts, or seeds on cereal and yogurt and add them to smoothies, baked goods, pancakes, and salads.
- Spread natural nut butter on whole-grain bread, crackers, or bagels, and use nut butter as a dip for fruit, such as apple slices and bananas.
- Snack on unsweetened dried fruit and nuts, such as raisins, dried plums, dried apricots, peanuts, and walnuts.
- Add chopped or sliced boiled eggs and avocado to salads and sandwiches.
- Add legumes (beans and peas) to soups, casseroles, and salads.
- If you can't cook, purchase affordable meals from Meals on Wheels or check into meals offered at a senior community center.

MyPlate for Older Adults

Fruits & Vegetables

Whole fruits and vegetables are rich in important nutrients and fiber. Choose fruits and vegetables with deeply colored flesh. Choose canned varieties that are packed in their own juices or low-sodium.

Healthy Oils

Liquid vegetable oils and soft margarines provide important fatty acids and some fat-soluble vitamins.

Herbs & Spices

Use a variety of herbs and spices to enhance flavor of foods and reduce the need to add salt.

Fluids

Drink plenty of fluids. Fluids can come from water, tea, coffee, soups, and fruits and vegetables.

Grains

Whole grain and fortified foods are good sources of fiber and B vitamins.

Dairy

Fat-free and low-fat milk, cheeses and yogurts provide protein, calcium and other important nutrients.

Protein

Protein rich foods provide many important nutrients. Choose a variety including nuts, beans, fish, lean meat and poultry.

Remember to Stay Active!

Tufts UNIVERSITY

JEAN MAYER USDA HUMAN NUTRITION RESEARCH CENTER ON AGING | HNRCA

AARP Foundation

USDA MyPlate and the other healthy eating patterns described in Chapter 3, but it is adapted slightly to best meet the needs of older adults.

This simple guide encourages you to choose several different categories of foods at every meal, which can help you take in a broader variety of vitamins, minerals, and other nutrients.

- **Make vegetables and fruits half of every meal.** These powerhouse foods are rich in vitamins, minerals, antioxidants, and other beneficial plant components that support health and activity.
- **Go for protein-rich foods.** Fish, chicken, turkey, eggs, lean red meat, legumes, natural nut butter, tofu, and dairy products, such as low-fat Greek yogurt and reduced-fat cheese should be a quarter of your meal.
- **Get help from whole grains.** Consume whole-wheat bread, brown rice, barley, rye crackers, and oatmeal to supply complex carbohydrates to help fuel your muscles, B vitamins to support metabolism, and fiber to help keep your digestive tract running smoothly. Smaller amounts of fortified refined grains, such as unsweetened fortified breakfast cereal, also can be included in your whole grains list.
- **Choose plant-based oils.** Used in small amounts, these oils (soybean, corn, canola, and olive oils) and soft spreads provide essential fatty acids (needed in small amounts) and some fat-soluble vitamins. Since the risk for high blood pressure increases with age, herbs and spices are recommended to enhance the flavor of foods, when needed, instead of salt.
- **Stay hydrated throughout the day.** Top choices are water, tea, and low-fat (1 percent) milk. You can include small amounts of coffee and small servings of 100 percent fruit juice, if desired. Soup also makes a substantial contribution to your fluid intake.

Taste Buds Change

In addition to poor eating habits, there are age-related factors that can impact food intake. The number of taste buds diminishes with age, decreasing the ability to taste sweet or salty, leaving foods tasting more sour or bitter. While it may be tempting to add salt and sugar to foods to compensate, both are linked to increased cardiovascular disease risk. Instead, experiment with the use of herbs and spices to boost flavor and enjoyment of foods.

Dental problems can make eating difficult. Get these issues addressed as soon as possible. If chewing is a problem, choose moist, soft foods, like stewed meats and tuna or egg salad for protein. Mash root vegetables like potatoes, yams, squashes, and more exotic choices like rutabaga, parsnip, or turnip. Purée or cream vegetables like spinach and enjoy fruit and veggie smoothies. These moist foods, with sauces and gravies, also help if medication side effects are causing dry mouth but watch out for acidic foods like tomato sauce and citrus, as these may irritate a dry mouth.

Constipation and stomach upset are common due to medication side effects and naturally slow digestion. Plenty of fiber-rich whole grains, fruits, and vegetables, along with increased fluid intake, can ease constipation. If a chronic upset stomach makes food unappetizing, try multiple small meals a day, experiment with different foods to see which are best tolerated, and work with your doctor and a registered dietitian to be sure you are getting enough calories and nutrients.

Changes in stomach-acid secretion and changes in the metabolism of foods can lead to vitamin B_{12} deficiency. Getting plenty of protein foods like dairy, eggs, meat, poultry, seafood, or fortified soy foods will provide your body with the B_{12} it needs.

The amount of water in the body decreases by approximately 15 percent between the ages of 20 and 80. This puts an older person at greater risk of dehydration from small losses of water. The ability to register thirst often declines as well. With age, the body's ability to concentrate urine decreases, and you may find yourself visiting the restroom more often. These changes increase the risk of dehydration in older adults. It's essential to make sure you are drinking enough, even if you don't feel thirsty.

Bone Health

Strong bones help you remain physically active and independent into old age. Resistance exercises help keep bones strong, but a ready supply of bone-building minerals and vitamins is also essential. Most minerals in your body are contained in your bones. In general, the denser this network of minerals is, the stronger your bones are and the more protection you have against fractures. Physically active people generally have greater bone-mineral density than those who are sedentary.

People reach peak bone mass around age 30. After that, your goal is to minimize losing bone mass as you age. Although both men and women are vulnerable to bone loss, hormonal changes in women speed up bone loss in the year or two before menopause and the five years or so after menopause.

Bone mass is greatly affected by nutrition. If you don't consume adequate calcium, your body pulls this mineral from your bones to supply your nerves and muscles with what they need. Vitamins D and K are also important in bone formation. Following a healthy eating pattern can help you get enough of all of them. (Sun exposure is also a strong source of vitamin D, but it isn't without risk. Discuss this with your physician.)

Dairy products are well-known as good sources of bone-building calcium, although the mineral also can be obtained from broccoli, kale, almonds, and calcium-fortified foods, such as orange juice, tofu, and milk substitutes.

Supplement if Needed

Supplements can be important to aging adults to make up nutritional inadequacies that often result from a reduced intake of food. A blood test can reveal which vitamins may be needed and how much to take. This should be done in consultation with your physician because taking too much of some can cause problems. Medications also need to be considered.

Meal-replacement drinks provide some fluids, vitamins, minerals, and protein. These drinks may be helpful to people too ill to prepare their own smoothie, but it's better to get nutrients from whole foods (or puréed whole foods). Be aware that these meal-replacement drinks can help people eat less regular food. Also be sure to check the nutrients label as some may be loaded with sugar.

Vitamin and mineral supplement pills like vitamin D, iron, or calcium may be necessary if you are unable to get enough of these nutrients from foods, but discuss what to use with your doctor. Research is conflicting. For example, there have been studies touting the benefits of vitamin D for muscle health, but results have been mixed. One study from Tuft's researchers reported that there may be some benefit to vitamin D supplementation for muscle function in certain segments of the population. But their trial did not show benefit for generally healthy community-dwelling older adults with moderately reduced vitamin D levels.

Multivitamins are unnecessary unless there are serious gaps in your diet that can't be addressed through modifying your eating patterns. Other supplements, such as herbal supplements, are largely unregulated, are not subject to Food & Drug Administration (FDA)

Dehydration Symptoms

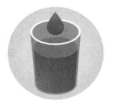
Thirst

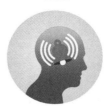
Headache

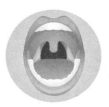
Dry mouth

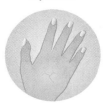
Dry skin

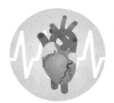
Rapid heartbeat

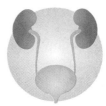
Decreased urination

© VectorMine | Dreamstime

Learn the symptoms of dehydration. As we grow older, our body might be a little slow in telling us we need hydration.

approval and could interact with medications (see "Safe Supplement Choices").

Considerations for Chronic Conditions

The benefits of healthy eating and regular exercise can be especially valuable to those with chronic conditions. In some cases, healthy lifestyle choices may reduce or eliminate the need for medications or reverse a condition entirely. It's always wise to discuss changes in dietary and exercise plans with your health-care provider. Your physician and health-care team are your allies and can help track progress and provide ideas for when you get stuck.

Easing Joint Pain

Achy joints, especially in your knees and hips, may keep you from wanting to move. But "motion is lotion" as physical therapists will attest. In addition to relieving pain, evidence indicates that exercise can help prevent or slow osteoarthritis damage. Some people especially benefit from simple stretches in the morning while still in bed. For example, open and close your hands, bend and straighten the knees, and gently twist the torso from side to side. If you have rheumatoid arthritis, exercise can help to relieve symptoms and improve day-to-day functioning. Yoga, in particular, can be quite helpful.

Activity trackers can help those with arthritis and other musculoskeletal issues increase physical activity. One study used wearable trackers like simple pedometers as well as more high-tech devices, such as a Fitbit. The study included 1,588 people with an average age of 55. The researchers found a significant increase in physical activity among users of activity trackers over a period of about 14 weeks.

The Arthritis Foundation recommends range-of-motion and flexibility exercises, coupled with aerobic and strength-training exercises. Walking and water exercises are particularly easy on the joints, and aquatic resistance training may be able to slow or even stop the progression of knee osteoarthritis. Other low-impact choices are cycling or using an elliptical machine.

High-impact activities like basketball should be limited and hard surfaces avoided. If you are new to exercise or unsure what's right for you, work with your doctor and/or a physical therapist to design an exercise plan for your needs.

Dietary changes may help control arthritis as well. A new study showed a relationship between diet and pain. A Mediterranean dietary pattern (see Chapter 3) is rich in foods that have been found to help control inflammation. The omega-3 fatty acids in fish and nuts; the antioxidants in fruits, vegetables, and beans; and the fiber in whole plant foods all have anti-inflammatory potential.

Some people report that nightshade vegetables (eggplant, tomatoes, peppers, and potatoes) make their arthritis pain worse. If you suspect this is the case for you, try cutting these foods out of your diet. If symptoms don't improve after two to four weeks, add them back in.

Enhancing Heart Health

If you have cardiovascular disease (CVD), such as atherosclerosis (hardening and narrowing of the arteries), heart failure, high blood pressure, or a history of a stroke or heart attack, diet and exercise can help improve or manage your condition.

Exercise can help control weight and improve CVD risk factors like high blood pressure and blood lipids (cholesterol). Regular physical activity also may reduce the need for medications. Exercise improves quality of life in CVD and makes it easier to perform self-care tasks.

Even so, there are precautions a person with CVD should take. In high-risk CVD, exercise may not be recommended.

While most people with CVD may be able to exercise on their own after seeking their doctor's guidance, your doctor may recommend you exercise under supervision of trained health personnel, such as at a cardiac-rehabilitation center if you are at a particularly high risk. Both aerobic and resistance training are generally recommended for people with CVD who have their doctor's approval to exercise.

A cool-down session immediately after exercise is especially important if you have heart issues, since most problems associated with exercise in CVD occur after exercise. Your doctor can tell you if any health conditions or medications you are on could cause problems with exercise.

Diet is key to controlling high blood pressure, keeping your arteries clear, and controlling heart failure. While the diet advice offered in Chapter 3 is a good guideline, some additional recommendations apply to certain cardiovascular issues. Everyone should limit saturated fat, but if you have high cholesterol, you should be especially vigilant. A reduced-sodium, high plant-food diet, like the Dietary Approaches to Stop Hypertension (DASH) plan described in Chapter 3, has been proven to improve blood pressure. People with heart failure should follow their doctor's or dietitian's sodium and fluid recommendations as closely as possible.

Improving for Diabetes

If you have type 2 diabetes or prediabetes, exercising and eating well are the best things you can do to help improve blood-sugar control, enhance insulin sensitivity (which makes your body's cells more responsive to insulin), and reduce CVD risk factors.

A combination of resistance training and aerobic exercise may be especially helpful in improving A1C—a blood test that measures average blood sugar over a period of three months—in people with type 2 diabetes. In some cases, a regular exercise program may even lead to your doctor being able to reduce your diabetes medication. New research suggests high-intensity interval training (HIIT) may be another exercise option useful in type 2 diabetes management or prevention (see Chapter 2).

In the short term, exercise can help lower blood sugar because in sustained moderate-exercise sessions muscles take up glucose at almost 20 times the normal rate. Additionally, exercising muscle can absorb glucose on its own, without the use of insulin, and muscle cells also become more responsive to the effects of insulin with exercise. Just a single exercise session may increase insulin sensitivity for up to two or three days (and you should exercise regularly to maintain this effect). So, you'll need less insulin to do the same job and you'll reduce surges in insulin that can contribute to heart disease, high blood pressure, and other health concerns.

If you take insulin or sulfonylurea medications, you could experience hypoglycemia (low blood sugar) during exercise if adjustments aren't made. Special precautions must be followed to ensure your blood sugar is in reasonable control before engaging in exercise, especially if you take insulin to control your blood sugar. Exercise performance seems to be best when blood sugar is maintained between 80 and 180 milligrams per deciliter.

Remember that the longer you have had diabetes, the more likely it is you have developed microvascular complications (diseases of the smallest blood vessels) that could impact your exercise program. If you have conditions like retinopathy (eye disease), peripheral neuropathy (nerve disease), and nephropathy (kidney disease), you may require certain precautions during exercise and/or the avoidance of certain kinds of physical activity. Your

Low Blood Sugar Warning Signs

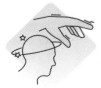

Shaky or dizzy

Blurry vision

Sweaty

Weak or tired

Upset or nervous

Headache

Hungry

© VectorMine | Dreamstime

Low blood sugar can affect people who don't have diabetes. It's important to learn the signs.

health-care team can assess your condition and determine what types of exercise are appropriate and whether any restrictions are needed.

Exercise for Osteoporosis

You can fight back against osteoporosis with good nutrition and physical activity and, in some cases, you may need to take bone-strengthening medications. In general, resistance training (two or three sessions per week) and weight-bearing aerobic activity (at least four sessions per week) are recommended to assist in maintaining and preventing bone loss. Resistance exercise causes muscle to contract against bone, and this stimulates the bone to become stronger and denser.

In 1994, Miriam Nelson, PhD, and her colleagues at Tufts University published a ground-breaking study showing that postmenopausal women (ages 50 to 70) who lifted weights twice a week for a year gained an average of 1 percent of their bone density, while those women who didn't exercise lost about 2 percent of their bone density, which is typical after menopause. Since then, other studies have confirmed that strength training is generally safe and can support bone health, even after menopause.

High-impact weight-bearing aerobic activity such as running or jumping rope may help improve bone density more quickly compared with low-impact activity, such as a brisk walk. High-impact aerobic activity isn't safe for everyone, though, so check with your health-care team first. Non-impact aerobic exercise, such as swimming, water aerobics, and bicycling, are good for your cardiovascular health but don't seem to place a sufficient load on the bone tissue to maintain or improve bone density.

If you have osteoporosis, get your physician's guidance and consult a physical therapist experienced in osteoporosis to discuss the best exercise program for you. A physical therapist also can assess kyphosis (an overly rounded back) and determine if there are exercises you should avoid. Expert instruction in correct technique for resistance training is especially important for those with poor bone health.

The same advice holds if you are frail or a fall risk. You're considered frail if you have three of these five criteria:

1. Poor muscle strength
2. Physical exhaustion
3. Low physical activity (sedentary lifestyle)
4. Slow walking speed
5. Unintentional weight loss

If you checked one or two, you may be at "pre-frailty," which means exercise may help you fight back. If you can slow the onset of frailty, you may reduce your risk of becoming disabled or losing your independence.

A Diet for Better Bones

The National Osteoporosis Foundation recommends you consume a well-balanced diet with plenty of dairy, fish, fruits, and vegetables. These foods are rich in calcium, vitamin D, and other nutrients that support bone health (see "Bone-Building Foods").

Beans contain calcium, magnesium, and other beneficial nutrients, but they also contain phytates, which block the absorption of calcium. To reduce the phytate level, soak beans in water for several hours, then drain. Wheat bran also contains phytates. Also be aware that very high-protein diets can cause the body to lose calcium.

High-sodium foods can cause your body to lose calcium and lead to bone loss. If you are eating packaged processed foods, check the Nutrition Facts label for sodium content. A food is considered high in sodium if a serving provides 20 percent or more for the percent Daily Value. Aim to get no more than 2,300 milligrams (mg) of sodium per day (1,500 mg if you have hypertension).

While foods like spinach, rhubarb, and beet greens do contain calcium, they also are high in oxalates, which bind with their calcium so it's less available to you. These foods are healthy choices, but not a good way to get calcium.

Caffeinated drinks (coffee, tea, some colas) and too much alcohol can contribute to bone loss. (Note: Less than three cups of coffee a day does not seem to be a problem.)

Eating a healthy diet that includes plenty of calcium-rich foods can compensate for any negative effects from the calcium-depleting foods in your diet, so don't hesitate to enjoy generally healthy choices, even if they are not the best for bone health.

Choose a Healthy Lifestyle

Personal hurdles will vary on this journey, but it's a rewarding path. It does require some willpower, as there will be hurdles. The brain's reward system is highly tuned to immediate gratification, it wants what it wants—*now*. It's a primitive system designed to help early *homo sapiens* hunt, gather, and have sex to continue the species.

Unfortunately, that same system can kick in when we think we can't survive without that greasy burger and fries or that extra helping of chocolate cake. On top of that, the industrial food complex purposely creates foods that induce cravings (namely high in fat, sugar, added colors, and that perfect crunch and melt). It's not easy to overcome these obstacles. But, with a few tools and some successes under your belt, you can do it. Next time you think you can't resist a craving, put time on your side by setting a timer for 10 minutes. If you still *really* want what you crave (food for example), enjoy half. Then wait again. Slowly building a time cushion

Bone-Building Foods

Calcium, magnesium, potassium, and vitamins D, C, and K are all important for bone health. If you eat a well-balanced diet with plenty of dairy, fish, fruits, and vegetables, you should get enough of the nutrients you need every day. This chart provides examples of some foods that supply bone-strengthening nutrients.

FOOD		NUTRIENT
DAIRY	• low-fat and non-fat milk, yogurt, and cheese	calcium
FISH	• canned sardines and salmon	calcium
	• fatty varieties such as salmon, mackerel, tuna, and herring	vitamin D
FRUITS AND VEGETABLES	• collard greens, turnip greens, kale, okra, Chinese cabbage, dandelion greens, mustard greens, and broccoli	calcium
	• spinach, beet greens, okra, artichokes, potatoes, sweet potatoes, and raisins	magnesium
	• tomatoes, raisins, spinach, papaya, oranges, orange juice, bananas, plantains, and prunes	potassium
	• red peppers, green peppers, oranges, grapefruit, broccoli, strawberries, and pineapples	vitamin C
	• dark-green leafy vegetables, such as kale, collard greens, spinach, mustard greens, turnip greens, and brussels sprouts	vitamin K
FORTIFIED FOODS	• calcium and vitamin D are sometimes added to certain brands of juices, breakfast foods, soy milk, rice milk, cereals, snacks, and breads	calcium vitamin D

Source: National Osteoporosis Foundation

can help separate craving from the real need to fuel your body.

Another strategy is imagining your future self. Is there something you really want to do in a few weeks or months? Take an adventure-travel hiking vacation, attend a grandchild's wedding, or master a pose in yoga class? Having a goal that's relevant and realistic and calling it to mind when you want to indulge in something unhealthy can help motivate you to stay on track. It doesn't matter what it is, so long as it matters to you.

Eating well and exercising offers opportunities to have more energy, better health, and greater enthusiasm for living. Remember, it's not about perfection. There's room for treats and pauses. A healthy lifestyle is about making wise choices the rule rather than the exception.

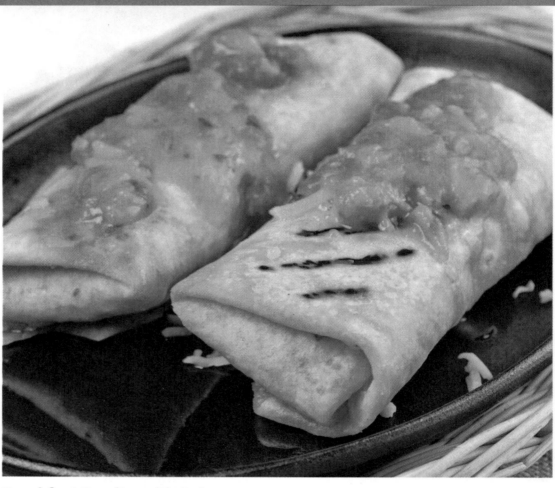

Breakfast Burrito with Salsa

Ingredients

4 large eggs
2 Tbsp frozen corn
1 Tbsp 1% milk
2 Tbsp diced red or green pepper
¼ cup minced onion
1 clove garlic, minced
1 Tbsp diced fresh tomatoes
1 tsp mustard*
¼ tsp hot pepper sauce (optional)
4 (8-inch) whole-wheat flour tortillas
½ cup prepared salsa**

* May use brown or Dijon mustard
  in place of yellow mustard.

** To reduce sodium content, choose
  low-sodium or no-salt-added salsa.

Steps

1. Preheat oven to 350°F.
2. In a large mixing bowl, blend the eggs, corn, milk, green peppers, onions, tomatoes, mustard, garlic, hot pepper sauce, and salt for 1 minute until eggs are smooth.
3. Pour egg mixture into a lightly oiled 9 x 9 inch baking dish and cover with foil.
4. Bake for 20–25 minutes until eggs are set and thoroughly cooked.
5. Place tortillas on microwave-safe plate, cover with paper towel, and microwave for 10–20 seconds until warm.
6. Cut baked egg mixture into 4 equal pieces; roll 1 piece of cooked egg in each tortilla.
7. Serve each burrito topped with 2 Tbsp of salsa.

Yield: 4 servings
Per serving: 233 calories, 9 g total fat, 3 g sat fat, 11 g protein, 29 g carbs, 4 g fiber, 3 g sugar, 491 mg sodium
Recipe (adapted): USDA Healthy Eating on a Budget
Photo: © Svetlana Foote | Dreamstime

Recipe Abbreviations

tsp = teaspoon
Tbsp = tablespoon
oz = ounces
lb = pound
g = grams
mg = milligrams

Barley, Pineapple, and Jicama Salad with Avocado

Ingredients

1 cup hulled (not pearled or flaked) barley

2 Tbsp fresh lime juice

¼ cup olive oil

¼ tsp ground cumin

¼ tsp salt

¼ tsp ground black pepper

6 cups watercress or 6 cups arugula, washed

1 medium jicama, peeled and grated

2 cups cubed pineapple
   (about ½ medium pineapple, peeled and cored)

2 large avocados, cubed

Steps

1. Bring barley and 3 cups water to a boil; reduce heat and simmer, covered, for 45–60 minutes, until liquid is absorbed and the grains are tender.
2. While barley is cooking, whisk together lime juice, olive oil, cumin, salt, and pepper.
3. In a large bowl, toss watercress or arugula with half of the dressing.
4. When barley is done cooking, drain off any excess liquid. Add barley, jicama, pineapple, and avocado to the greens along with the rest of the dressing; toss gently to combine.

Yield: 6 servings
Per serving: 349 calories, 17 g total fat, 2 g sat fat, 6 g protein, 48 g carbs, 15 g fiber, 8 g sugar, 116 mg sodium
Recipe (adapted) and photo: Oldways, oldwayspt.org

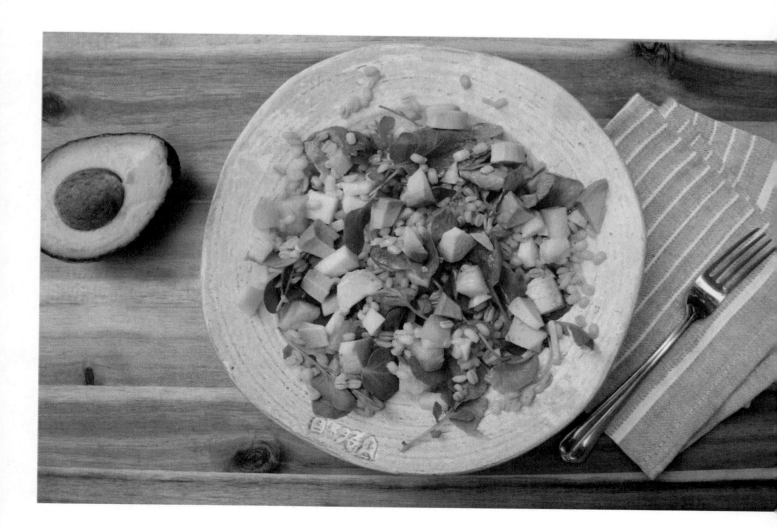

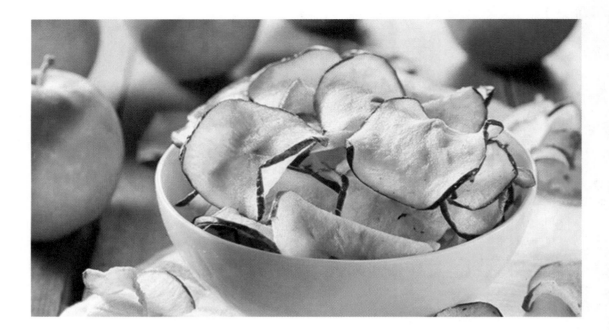

Baked Apple Chips

Ingredients
- 4 large apples (any variety, unpeeled)
- 2 tsp cinnamon
- 1 Tbsp granulated sugar

Steps
1. Slice apples horizontally into very thin rounds, using a sharp knife or mandolin. Remove any seeds that do not fall out as you cut.
2. Combine cinnamon and sugar.
3. Lay the apple slices in a single layer on a baking sheet lined with parchment paper; sprinkle lightly with the cinnamon sugar.
4. Bake apple slices at 250°F for 1 hour, flip slices, and bake for an additional hour (2 hours total). Chips will continue to crisp up as they cool.

Yield: 8 servings
Per serving: 66 calories, 0 g total fat, 0 g sat fat, 0 g protein, 17 g carbs, 3 g fiber, 13 g sugar, 0 mg sodium
Recipe (adapted) and photo: American Institute for Cancer Research, aicr.org

Veggie Pad Thai

Ingredients

Sauce

1 Tbsp fish sauce
2 Tbsp rice vinegar
1 Tbsp reduced-sodium soy sauce or tamari

1 Tbsp honey
¼ cup lime juice (juice of 1–2 limes)

Pad Thai

8 oz wide, flat rice noodles
   (preferably brown rice noodles), uncooked
1 Tbsp olive, sesame, or canola oil, divided
8 oz extra-firm tofu, drained and cut into ½-inch cubes
2 large eggs
½ yellow onion, chopped
3 cloves garlic, minced
1 head of broccoli, cut into small florets

1 zucchini, spiralized (or sliced into thin, long strips)
1 cup snap peas
2 carrots, grated
1 cup mung bean sprouts
¼ cup fresh basil, chopped
¼ cup fresh cilantro, chopped
Crushed red pepper, to taste

Garnishes

2 Tbsp peanuts, chopped

Lime wedges

Steps

1. In a small bowl, whisk together all the sauce ingredients; set aside.
2. Prepare the noodles according to package instructions. Drain noodles and set aside.
3. In a large skillet, heat 1½ teaspoons of oil over medium-high heat.
4. Add tofu to skillet and sauté about 3 minutes, or until just getting golden brown. Rotate the pieces to get a golden color on all sides. Move tofu to edge of pan.
5. Crack eggs into pan, break yolks with spatula, and scramble eggs until just cooked through (about 1 minute). Set the egg and tofu aside on a plate.
6. Add remaining oil to pan. Add onion and garlic to pan and sauté 1–2 minutes, or until just translucent.
7. Add broccoli, zucchini, snap peas, and carrots; sauté until they are just fork-tender and still bright in color, about 3 minutes.
8. Add noodles, sauce, tofu, and eggs to the pan. Gently mix everything together so the flavors combine and the noodles can soak up the sauce. Add half of the bean sprouts, basil, and cilantro, mix gently, and remove from heat.
9. Serve topped with remaining bean sprouts, basil, and cilantro, peanuts, and lime wedges on the side.

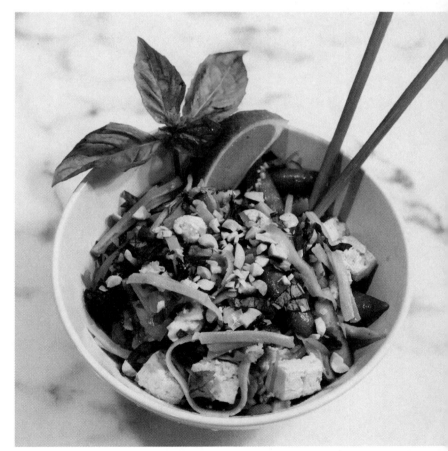

Yield: 4 servings (1½-2 cups each)
Per serving: 475 calories, 13 g total fat, 2 g sat fat, 21 g protein, 74 g carbs, 9 g fiber, 13 g sugar, 647 mg sodium
Recipe (adapted) and photo: American Institute for Cancer Research, aicr.org

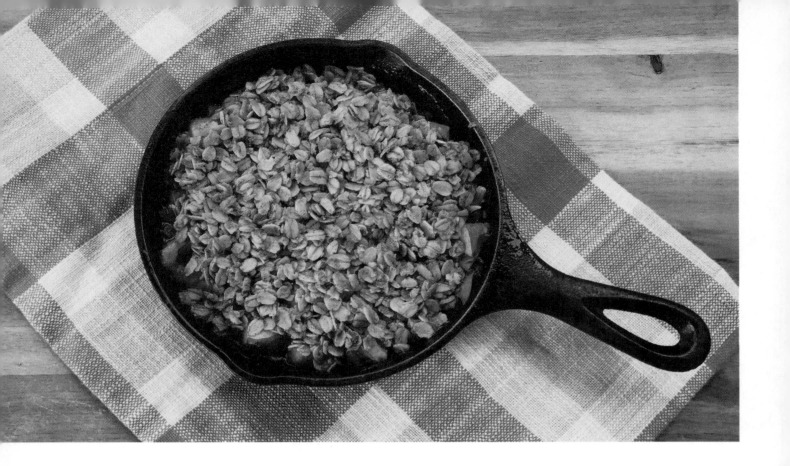

Easy Peach Crisp

Ingredients

- 1 Tbsp plus 1 tsp olive oil, divided
- ½ cup rolled oats
- 1 tsp sugar
- ¼ tsp cinnamon
- 2 cups peaches, diced (or apples, berries, etc.)
- Vanilla frozen yogurt (optional)

Steps

1. Preheat oven to 350°F. Grease a 6½-inch cast iron skillet with 1 tsp olive oil.
2. In a small bowl, toss oats with cinnamon, sugar, and remaining olive oil.
3. Put fruit in skillet and top with oat mixture. Bake for 35 minutes, until fruit is bubbly and oats are golden brown.
4. Let cool for 5–10 minutes; top with a scoop of vanilla frozen yogurt, if desired. (Caution: The skillet will be very hot.)

Yield: 2 servings
Per serving, without yogurt: 209 calories, 11 g total fat, 1 g sat fat, 6 g protein, 34 g carbs, 6 g fiber, 14 g sugar, 1 mg sodium
Recipe (adapted) and photo: Oldways, oldwayspt.org

WALL PUSH-UPS

- Extend your arms and place your hands on the wall at shoulder width.

- Brace your abs and extend/lengthen your spine.

- Bend your elbows and slowly lower your upper body toward the wall.

- Hold for 1–2 seconds, then push back until your arms are straight.

- 8–10 reps, 2–3 sets.

    Where to Feel the Effort: Back of arms, shoulder blades, abs.

    Variation: The progression of this exercise is: 1) wall push-ups for beginners, 2) countertop push-ups using a table, desk, countertop, or other sturdy object for intermediate-level exercisers, and 3) traditional push-ups performed on a mat for those who are able.

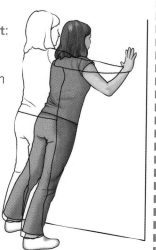

SEMI-SITS

- Stand in front of a chair, feet hip-width apart.

- Brace your abs.

- Slowly begin to sit down in a sturdy chair, but just touch the chair seat lightly before returning to a standing position. (Think about letting your pants crease but not your shirt.)

- Work up to 8–10 repetitions, 2–3 sets.

    Where to Feel the Effort: Buttocks, thighs.

    Variation: Lower your buttocks just a few inches instead of going far enough to touch the chair seat. Restrict the number of repetitions to 4–5 and the number of sets to 1–2.

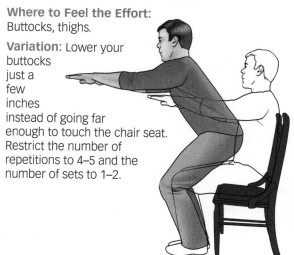

LUNGES

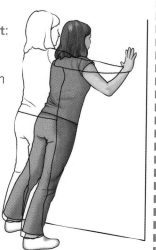

- Start standing with feet hip width apart. Step forward 12 inches.

- As you step, sit back into the pose shown. Imagine the position "on your mark, get set."

- Your chest should line up over the hips, and the knee should line up over your shoelaces.

- Let the back heel come up off the floor.

- Push up through your whole foot to standing position. You should be able to wiggle your toes in your shoes when the foot is forward.

- Work up to 8–10 repetitions and 2–3 sets for each leg.

- Increase the load by holding 3- to 8-pound dumbbells in each hand.

    Where to Feel the Effort: Thighs, buttock of front leg.

    Variation: Reduce the number of repetitions to 4–5 and the number of sets to 1–2 until you begin to get stronger.

    NOTE: If you feel strain in your knees, use resistance bands. Your mechanics need tweaking. A physical therapist can help you feel the muscles of your thighs and buttocks but not knee strain.

SINGLE LEG STAND

- Stand with your feet slightly apart, head up. With your interior hand holding the chair for balance and your exterior hand on your outer hip, brace your abdomen, tighten your buttocks, and lift your outer leg off the floor until your knee is parallel with your hip.

- Hold for 5–10 seconds.

- Think about keeping your waistline level and your front pockets (pelvis) square to the front.

- Work up to balancing without your hand on the chair for 30–60 seconds.

- Change positions and repeat movement with the opposite leg.

- 3–5 repetitions on each side.

    Where to Feel the Effort: Maintaining balance without holding onto a chair.

    Variation: Limit the time balancing to 3–5 seconds.

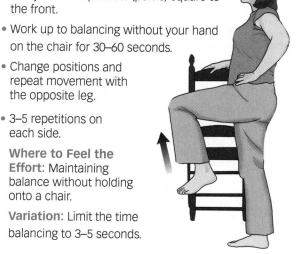

Exercise Illustrations by Alayna Paquette

GLOSSARY

A1C: A test that measures a person's average blood glucose level over the past two to three months. Also called hemoglobin A1C or glycosylated hemoglobin.

aerobic exercise: Physical activity that increases the intake and use of oxygen and improves the cardiovascular and respiratory systems. Sometimes called endurance exercise, it includes brisk walking, running or jogging, and cycling.

body mass index (BMI): A measure that combines your weight and height to assess whether you are a healthy weight, overweight, or obese: Weight in pounds / (height in inches x height in inches) x 703. A BMI of 18.5 to 24.9 is considered healthy weight; 25 to 29.9 is considered overweight, and 30 or higher is considered obese.

cardiovascular disease (CVD): A class of diseases that involve the heart or blood vessels. Includes coronary artery disease, heart disease, stroke, heart failure, and more.

cognition: Conscious intellectual activity, such as thinking and memory, orientation, language, judgment, and problem solving.

core muscles: The muscles of the abdomen, lower back, shoulder girdle, and hips.

coronary artery disease: Blockage of one or more arteries that supply blood to the heart, usually due to atherosclerosis (hardening of the arteries).

endurance exercise: Also called aerobic exercise.

free radical: A highly reactive atom or compound produced through normal metabolism or from environmental toxins, such as cigarette smoke and air pollutants. Free radicals damage cell membranes, DNA, proteins, and other molecules in the body. They are neutralized by antioxidants.

free weights: Dumbbells, barbells, or kettlebells, for example, used in resistance/strength exercise training.

glucose: A simple sugar used by the body as a source of energy that is the product of the breakdown of more complex carbohydrates.

glycemic index: A system that ranks foods on a scale from 1 to 100 based on their effect on blood-sugar levels.

glycogen: The form of glucose stored in the liver and muscles.

heart failure: A chronic, progressive disease in which the heart muscle weakens and can no longer pump blood well enough to meet the body's needs.

heart rate: The number of times your heart beats in one minute (pulse).

high-impact aerobic exercise: Physical activity that results in a heart rate of approximately 80 to 85 percent of maximum, and in which there is a greater impact on bones and joints.

high-intensity interval training (HIIT): Exercise that involves short bursts of intense activity followed by brief recovery periods.

insulin: A hormone released by the pancreas that causes cells to take up sugar (glucose) from the bloodstream to use and store for energy. Insulin is important in carbohydrate, fat, and protein metabolism.

insulin resistance: The body's inability to efficiently use the insulin it produces, which is linked to obesity and physical inactivity and occurs in type 2 diabetes.

kyphosis: A curving of the spine that causes a bowing or rounding of the back, which leads to a hunchback or slouching posture.

lipid: A word used to encompass many different kinds of fats or fat-soluble molecules, including cholesterol, triglycerides, and free fatty acids.

low-impact aerobic exercise: Physical activity in which there is a less-demanding cardiovascular effort and in which one foot is always in contact with the ground or surface.

maximum heart rate: The heart rate achieved at near an individual's maximum oxygen uptake. Estimated as approximately 220 beats per minute minus a person's age.

metabolic syndrome: Having three or more of these conditions: high triglycerides, low HDL (good) cholesterol, high blood pressure, elevated blood glucose, and a large waist circumference (abdominal obesity). Metabolic syndrome is associated with insulin resistance and an increased risk of diabetes and cardiovascular disease.

osteoarthritis: A joint disease characterized by the degeneration of cartilage and the underlying bone (also called "arthritis").

osteoporosis: A disease that causes a loss of bone density, causing the bones to become weak and brittle.

power: The ability to generate force as fast as possible (a product of strength and speed).

prediabetes: A condition in which blood sugar (glucose) levels are higher than normal but are not high enough for a diagnosis of diabetes. People with prediabetes are at increased risk for developing type 2 diabetes and for heart disease and stroke.

phytochemicals (also called phytonutrients): Compounds in plants that provide flavor, aroma, and color, and protect the plant from microbes and environmental damage. When consumed by humans, phytochemicals are believed to promote health and prevent disease. Many phytochemicals are antioxidants.

repetition (rep): The single act of lifting or moving a part of the body against resistance.

resistance bands: Elastic bands that act as resistance against movement during resistance training.

resistance training: A form of exercise that involves movement or attempted movement against resistance (or load). Also called strength training.

sarcopenia: Age-related loss of muscle mass and strength.

set: A group of consecutive repetitions (reps) of an exercise movement, without rest.

strength training: A form of exercise that involves movement or attempted movement against resistance (or load). Also called resistance training.

target heart rate zone: A heart rate range of approximately 50 to 75 percent of maximum heart rate, which is generally the target for aerobic conditioning.

triglycerides: A form of fat found in food, fat tissue, and the bloodstream. Elevated triglycerides in the bloodstream are a risk factor for heart disease.

type 1 diabetes: An autoimmune condition in which the body's immune system attacks insulin-producing beta cells in the pancreas and destroys them. As the pancreas stops producing insulin, blood sugar levels rise.

type 2 diabetes: Occurs when the pancreas does not produce enough insulin and/or the body's cells become resistant to insulin and causes increases in blood sugar levels.

vegan: A diet that eliminates all animal products, including dairy, eggs, and honey.

vegetarian: A diet that eliminates meat, but still may include dairy and eggs. Vegetarians who consume fish are called pescatarians.

weight training: Exercise in which a person lifts or moves weights to gain muscle strength or endurance. Also called resistance training or strength training.

Associations

Academy of Nutrition and Dietetics
eatright.org
800-877-1600

American Academy of Physical Medicine and Rehabilitation
847-737-6000
aapmr.org

AARP
888-687-2277
aarp.org

American College of Sports Medicine
317-637-9200
acsm.org

American Diabetes Association
800-342-2383
diabetes.org

American Heart Association
800-242-8721
heart.org

American Physical Therapy Association
800-999-2782
apta.org or moveforwardpt.com

American Society for Nutrition
240-428-3650
nutrition.org

Arthritis Foundation
404-872-7100
arthritis.org

Dietary Guidelines for Americans (2020-2025)
240-453-8280
dietaryguidelines.gov

Gerontological Society of America
202-842-1275
geron.org

National Association of Area Agencies on Aging
202-872-0888
n4a.org

National Council on Aging
571-527-3900
ncoa.org

National Heart, Lung and Blood Institute
877-645-2448
nhlbi.nih.gov

National Institute of Diabetes and Digestive and Kidney Diseases
800-860-8747
niddk.nih.gov

National Institute on Aging
800-222-2225
nia.nih.gov/health

National Osteoporosis Foundation
800-231-4222
nof.org

National Strength & Conditioning Association
800-815-6826
nsca.com

Physical Activity Guidelines for Americans
240-453-8280
health.gov/paguidelines

President's Council on Fitness, Sports & Nutrition
240-276-9567
fitness.gov

YMCA of the USA
800-872-9622
ymca.net

U.S. Food and Drug Administration
888-463-6332
fda.gov

Cookbooks

Here are some cookbooks to consider adding to your kitchen.

Eat to Beat Disease, William W. Li, MD (Hachette Books, 2019)

The China Study Quick & Easy Cookbook: Cook Once, Eat All Week with Whole Food, Plant-Based Recipes by LeAnne Campbell, PhD, (BenBella Books, 2018)

The Complete Month of Meals Collection (American Diabetes Association, 2017)

The Pescetarian Plan: The Vegetarian + Seafood Way to Lose Weight and Love Your Food Cookbook by Janis Jibrin and Sidra Forman (Ballantine Books, 2014)

Grill It, Braise It, Broil It: And 9 Other Easy Techniques for Making Healthy Meals by the American Heart Association (Harmony, 2015)

Joy of Cooking: 2019 Edition Fully Revised and Updated by Irma S. Rombauer (Scribner, 2019)

Mark Bittman's Kitchen Matrix: More Than 700 Simple Recipes and Techniques to Mix and Match for Endless Possibilities by Mark Bittman (Clarkson Potter, 2015)

The New American Heart Association Cookbook, 9th Edition (Harmony, 2019)

You Can Have It! More than 125 Decadent, Diabetes-Friendly Recipes by Devin Alexander (American Diabetes Association, 2018)

Online Recipe Sources

If you don't see a "recipes" link on the home page of these websites, simply type "healthy recipes" in the search box.

American Diabetes Association My Food Advisor
diabetesfoodhub.org

American Heart Association
heart.org

American Institute for Cancer Research
aicr.org

Fruits & Veggies—More Matters, Produce for Better Health Foundation
fruitsandveggies.org

Oldways
oldwayspt.org

Health & Nutrition Letter
Tufts University
nutritionletter.tufts.edu

Whole Grains Council
wholegrainscouncil.org

Exercise Books

Choosing the Strong Path: Reversing the Downward Spiral of Aging by Fred Bartlit, Steven Droullard, and Marni Boppart (Greenleaf Book Group Press, 2018)

Empowered Aging: Expert Advice on Staying Healthy, Vital and Active by Sharkie Zartman (Spoilers Press, 2018)

The Joy of Movement, Kelly McGonigal, PhD (Avery/Penguin Random House, 2019)

End Everyday Pain for 50+: A 10-Minute-a-Day Program of Stretching, Strengthening and Movement to Break the Grip of Pain by Dr. Joseph Tiere (Ulysses Press, 2016)

Free Online Exercise and Nutrition Resources

choosemyplate.gov: Provides practical information to help consumers build healthier diets. Includes resources and tools for dietary assessment and nutrition education.

consumerlab.com: Provides independent test results, reviews, ratings, and comparisons of vitamins, supplements, herbal and nutrition products.

ewg.org: The Environmental Working Group is a nonpartisan, nonprofit organization that conducts research and education about the environment and food to enable people to make safer and more informed purchasing decisions.

http://tiny.cc/NIA-NIHExercise: The latest from the National Institute on Aging on how exercise and physical activity can help keep you healthy as you age. The website is filled with exercise tips, tracking tools, and ways to stay motivated for life.

doyogawithme.com: Hundreds of free streaming videos offering yoga for all levels.

silversneakers.com: Free access to gyms, classes, and more.

sparkpeople.tv: Free workout videos of all types for all levels. Allows you to search for the length, type, and level you want.